$2.50

A MATTER OF TIMING

A MATTER OF TIMING

Alzheimer's — A Carer's Journey

Audrey Brown

The Book Guild Ltd
Sussex, England

The Book Guild Ltd
25 High Street,
Lewes, Sussex

First published 1998
© Audrey Brown, 1998
Set in Times
Typesetting by Raven Typesetters, Chester

Printed in Great Britain by
Bookcraft (Bath) Ltd, Avon

A catalogue record for this book is
available from the British Library

ISBN 1 85776 331 9

CONTENTS

Memory holds the whole of our past life and experience.
Its loss is greater than the loss of any of our senses. Anon.

Footfalls echo in the memory,
Down the passage we did not take,
Towards the door we never opened. *T.S. Eliot*

I've a grand memory for forgetting. *R.L. Stevenson*

When they begin the beguine ... it brings back a memory ever-green. *Cole Porter*

A memory of yesterday's pleasures. A fear of tomorrow's dangers. *John Donne*

There is only now.
The past is what we remember of what went on before.
The future is speculation of what may happen.
The only reality is the present.
> And happiness is the pursuit – not of future rewards –
> But the perfection of the moment. *Brian Redhead*

I am. Yet what I am none cares or knows.
My friends forsake me like a memory lost. *John Clare*

I know about Alzheimer's from the outside.
What a great deal more there is to learn from the inside. Anon.

I think – therefore I am. (*Cogito, ergo sum.*) *René Descartes*

FOREWORD

Few of us care too much about carers, do we? They're 'jolly good' to look after their disabled charges, of course, but have we any idea what their role entails? In the strange world of Alzheimer's, I suspect that most of us are as clueless about the emotions, the stresses, the desperation of the carers as we are about the illness itself.

Audrey Brown is a carer. And since I first met her, I have come to understand just a little of what she has been through in caring for her beloved Stan.

Where does she find the reserves of limitless patience, the physical and spiritual energy, the staying power, the good humour?

She is a remarkable woman; this is a remarkable book ... and not only for its insight into the painful discovery and experience of a partner's irreparable tragedy, but also for the way it reflects the making, since childhood, of its very special author.

Audrey Brown's account of life that began in a Lancashire family home with an outside loo and a tin bath brings tears and laughter in equal measure through a deceptively simple style and language.

My most lasting image of Audrey and Stan together was in their Worcester bungalow, she playing the piano, he whistling a quite different tune, his hands clasped in front of his happy face as though applauding their joint performance.

You couldn't help smiling. Even if there was also a tear running down your cheek.

Michael Barratt

INTRODUCTION

I suppose it started when I was born – this timing business I mean! I got it wrong then and I have been getting it wrong ever since. I should have been a January baby but I couldn't wait that long – I couldn't even wait until Christmas. 'Mrs Ellis,' said Doctor McCready, 'I think we may have problems – I think we should get you into the maternity home straight away.' My mother pulled herself up to her full height – all five feet nothing of her – took a deep breath and said, 'I'm ready.'

But I wasn't! Now that I knew everyone had been alerted, I went on a go-slow strike that lasted for five days – five long, exhausting and horribly painful days – at least that's what I have been told. Five days for everyone to get anxious and flustered, worried and tired. Five days of probing and pushing – until finally, loudly protesting and just one week before Christmas, I was born. What a stupid time to choose! Even to this day – and I have almost reached my three-score years and ten – I still get upset when my birthday and Christmas get confused. 'Happy Birthday!' says donor number one, handing me a parcel wrapped in Christmas paper. 'This is for Christmas as well. Please yourself when you open it.' 'Happy Birthday,' says number two. 'You'll have to wait till Christmas for your present.' Even worse are the parcels that arrive with no indication as to whether they are for birthday, Christmas or both. Shall I have the excitement on my birthday or wait until Christmas? By my age you would think I would have become reconciled to all of it but I still feel cheated. My birthday is always when Christmas preparations are at their height and I feel it is just a hiccup in all those preparations. Probably best forgotten altogether.

Anyway, here I was, one week before Christmas – and with the consensus of opinion that it possibly had not been worth all the effort. My poor, darling mother was very ill and I was a wreck and not expected to survive. I had arrived with a broken arm, a big gash on my neck, breathing problems, jaundice – and a very dim view of the outside world. But we were survivors, my mother and I – and from the start had a wonderful relationship that stood the test of time.

'Time' – there's that word again. I wish I could get it right – just once. All my life I have been far too early or extremely late. I imagine it will be the same with this book. Everyone is supposed to have at least one book in them. I have been cajoled, chivvied – even threatened – to write mine. So here goes. Mistimed, as always, but hopefully better late than never. It won't be an easy book to write – Alzheimer's disease is a difficult subject. At the moment I'm not even sure just how I am going to tackle it. My hope is that it will reach the hearts and minds of all who read it. I want it to be a true and honest account of a very ordinary couple and how Alzheimer's crept slowly and relentlessly into our lives and affected every aspect of those lives. Everything I write about will be real – real events, real people, real feelings, real thoughts. I may change the names of some of the people, even some of the places, but everything will be exactly as it happened. Inevitably there will be sadness but I hope I can also convey the wonder and joy of those fleeting moments of togetherness and the many happy moments that one of us, at least, remembers and savours.

PART ONE

THE SUNSHINE YEARS

1

Fun and Lessons

'Hello, Mum, I'm home!' Dishevelled and out of breath after my dash from school, I raced up the back street, into the backyard and through the door into the kitchen.

'Hello, love.' Mum was there as usual. Mum was always there. It never crossed my mind that she would be anywhere else. But even if she had just popped to the corner shop or to a neighbour's, the door would not be locked. It never was.

From the outside our house was just like the rest, a tiny terraced house with just four rooms – kitchen, living room and two bed-rooms – no bathroom and no toilet. That was in the backyard together with a coalplace and – a bit of one-upmanship – a small lean-to greenhouse which was Dad's pride and joy. And, in case you are wondering, the tin bath, to be used only on Fridays, was suspended from a large hook fixed into the outside wall.

The backstreet was like hundreds of others in the town – narrow, lit at night by just one gas lamp and paved with uneven and, at times, very slippery cobblestones. The front, though, was something special. We had a garden! Narrow, because our house was narrow, but very long with a little paved area outside the front door where we could sit when the weather was kind. A long path led to a garden gate and the narrow pavement outside. Where the street should have been was just long grass and nettles, rosebay willowherb, daisies, dandelions – and hen pens!

In summer the garden was magic. Clematis framed the front doorway. There was the perfume and colour of carefully tended roses. And there were the annuals, all grown from seed in the tiny

3

greenhouse and never failing to provide an astonishing kaleido-scope of colour that was unsurpassed.

The view beyond the garden was also magic. Our house was high above the main town and we could look over the tall mill chimneys towards the moors – towards Haworth and Brontë country. In the opposite direction, out on a limb away from the main Pennine chain, was my very favourite hill – Pendle Hill – set amid real Lancashire witches' landscape. A vast area with its own special magic, rugged and majestic, like nowhere else on earth. I loved it all!

'Well then?' Mum stopped peeling potatoes, perched herself on one of the kitchen stools and pointed to the other. 'Sit down and let's hear all about it.'

I tried to sound cheerful. 'It's all right, I suppose. It's big – I kept getting lost.'

'So – what did you do all day?'

'I – we – all the new ones went into the hall. We were there for ages and we were told our form number. I thought we would be in One-something or other but we're all in Form Three. We're some-thing called "unstreamed". I'm in Three C. We've got a form master, too. His name is Mr Duerden but everybody calls him Dicky Dubbin. That's it.'

'Yes – and then? Come on, what else did you do? You must have done something else.'

Mum was in one of her persistent moods. I just wished she would leave me alone. I'd had a horrible day. The grammar school was so huge and I felt so lonely. I didn't know anybody. There were a few others from my junior school but they were all fourth years and I was a mere third year – and they ignored me. Yes, I'd got my timing wrong again. I was still not quite ten years old but I had taken and passed my scholarship a year early. My parents were so proud. They had had to use the holiday money to buy my school uniform and a brand new leather satchel. We'd only had a day trip to Blackpool during the summer. They tried to make it very special but I felt sad. Sad about them having to miss a proper holiday, sad about leaving my school friends behind and saddest of all about not quite finishing the cane basket I'd been making which was quite the best thing I'd ever done. Just one more lesson

4

and it would have been finished. 'We will finish them all next term,' Miss Whittaker had said, quite forgetting that I wouldn't be there. I wanted it so badly but I was afraid to say anything to her. Why, oh why did I have to leave my beautiful basket and all my special friends behind just to go to that stupid school? I really had got my timing wrong.

I don't know how long my misery lasted. It wasn't just school either. It was when I got home from school too. I was suddenly 'different'. The children who lived nearby didn't call for me to play out any more; they went off without me to all our secret places – down the delph, our favourite hiding place, round the back of the garages and through the broken railings into the mill yard. I didn't feel any different – but I was no longer one of them. I rushed through my homework and then had to play on my own in the backyard. Perhaps skipping – 'One, two, three alaira, I saw my sister Sarah, sitting on a band-alera, eating chocolate biscuits.' And 'Salt, mustard, vinegar, pepper' is so boring unless the rope is turned by others getting faster and faster all the time. I played hop-scotch and tried to beat my own record. I played top and whip, but my chalk patterns didn't matter any more – I couldn't compare them with those of my friends. Ball games were played against the house wall – I invented lots of variations. Soon I began to play competitively with my two imaginary friends but somehow I always won! They were lovely friends, Princess Elizabeth and Princess Margaret Rose – not many people know that the future Queen and her sister once played in our backyard! I did 'dips' to decide who would have first 'go' with the ball – again I always won. 'Ip, dip, pen and ink. Who made that great big stink? I think it was you!' Oh, how I missed my real friends – Una, Rosie, Rene, Mabel, Theresa and Jean, and the boys Leslie, Chris and Paul. It was the first time I had encountered such inverted snobbery.

Gradually, as I became more used to my new school and a very different daily way of life, school began to appeal to me more and more. I suppose it is common sense when you think about it. Everything that you can take in your stride becomes routine and no longer holds any terrors. Lessons fitted into that category. I was eager to learn, I was a conformist and I was one of those lucky people able to sort out the essential details for passing exams. That

5

part of my life soon faded into insignificance and the details were stored away into a special compartment of my brain labelled 'Done it. Finished with it. Now forget all about it'.

The hardest thing of all had been to keep pretending to Mum and Dad that everything was fine, until suddenly, I'm not quite sure when, I didn't have to pretend any more. Life again was quite wonderful. School held no more worries for me – I had found my feet, I knew what I was doing and I was thoroughly enjoying the challenge. I had new friends. My best buddies, Marian and Jean, were simply great. And then there was Amy, who was a bit of a snob really, because her father was 'in banking', but still good fun. And Doreen, too clever for her own good but great for telling us the answers for our Latin homework. We ignored the boys in our form and they avoided us like the plague. At the end of the first year, I sailed through the exams and was placed in the top form (Four A) in year two.

The bits of school that I still remember are those bits that were not routine. They, too, slot quite neatly into a couple of compartments in my brain labelled 'This isn't fair', and 'I really shouldn't be doing this, but isn't it fun?' In the first slot was my experience with the headmistress, a certain Miss Cliffe, who struck terror into the hearts of all who crossed her path. Our first meeting was in the English literature lesson. Her reputation had gone before her, so with sinking hearts we filed silently into the room, took our places without even a sound of scraping seats and waited, not even daring to glance at one another. Miss Cliffe, seated behind a table apparently engrossed in her book and unaware of our presence, totally ignored us.

We waited ... we began to risk a surreptitious glance at each other. One brave soul began to fidget, another gave a little cough ... we waited. Eventually, slowly and deliberately, the book was closed and placed carefully to one side. The head was raised and the spectacles were moved down to the end of her nose. A pair of steely grey eyes slowly inspected each and every one of us – we froze. 'So,' her voice was as hard as steel, cold and penetrating – 'So this is what you do in my lesson, is it?' We sat silent and waited. 'Let me tell you now. This is *not* what you do in my lesson. You have wasted at least five minutes of valuable study time.

6

What have you done?'

She pierced one unfortunate boy with her stare until, red-faced and uncomfortable he managed to stammer 'We...we've...w...w...wasted time.'

After what seemed an eternity, the voice continued. 'You have wasted time – you will never, I repeat *never*, do that again. In future, you will come into the room, take out your book and read. You will savour every word of what you read – you will learn to appreciate the skill and the style of the author, and you will not, I repeat *not* waste time again...'

Having established her authority, she then began the first of what became the most boring lessons imaginable. Starting at the beginning of our new study book, *A Tale of Two Cities*, which we renamed out of sheer boredom *A Sale of Two Titties*, we took turns in reading a paragraph each until everyone had had a turn. And that was supposed to be English literature! She then told us what we had read – the humour, the pathos, the sarcasm, the figures of speech, the innuendos. We weren't allowed to discuss or think for ourselves. She was the one who would dictate and she would be obeyed.

Even worse, she had her own way of addressing us, which was so insulting and hurtful to anyone who did not fit into her snobbish categorisation of acceptable society. Amy, the bank manager's daughter, was always addressed by Christian name only. 'Amy, dear,' she would say and smile sweetly. Sheila's father was a schoolteacher – not bad, I suppose, but he had not risen very far up the scale – so Sheila got her full name and no smile. 'Sheila Fielding, continue reading, please.' As for me, my father was working class. He was a nobody. When it came to my turn, I simply got surname only. 'Ellis,' she would say, 'continue.' There was no 'please' and certainly no smile. I had never felt so hurt and humiliated.

In a funny sort of way, I eventually got my own back, even though it was completely unintentional. I read the letters 'g-a-o-l' as 'goal'. Well, how was I supposed to know that there was an alternative spelling for 'jail'? The whole class roared with laughter and even Miss Cliffe momentarily lost control. Later, though, when I referred to Job, the prophet as 'job – a task, employment',

7

like Queen Victoria, she was not amused, and I was punished for being insolent.

Also in the 'This isn't fair' category was a happening which was a total injustice. It was the exams at the end of year one which determined the 'streaming' for year two. We were well spaced out in the hall and I felt to be doing all right. During the physics exam I became aware of the boy at the next desk trying to attract my attention. Through sign-language I realised he needed a ruler and I quite openly passed one to him. We were spotted by the invigilator. We were given no chance to explain and our papers were cancelled. I was devastated by this – it really was most unfair. As it happened it made no difference to my placing in the top form in year two – I came third out of the whole of the first-year pupils. But what hurt was the injustice of the whole thing and the realisation that with even low marks for physics, I would have probably been in first place and would then have received the form prize, an honour that was denied me.

Into the 'It's great fun' compartment were the beginnings of my rebellious streak, flouting authority and allowing myself to be led astray by the more habitual offenders. In chemistry lessons I found it great fun to stick peanuts into the end of a compass point and then roast them on the Bunsen burners. Perhaps I wasn't quite as good as the rest but, for whatever reason, I was the one who got caught and had to stand on a high stool out in the corridor, much to my chagrin.

French lessons were a hoot. Mrs Thompson had an alarm clock which she set to ring just before the school bell so that she had time to set our homework. We discovered it was faulty – the alarm could not be stopped, the mechanism had to be allowed to run down. That was why it was only wound half a turn. Until we sabotaged it! We set it to go off just minutes into the lesson and wound it fully. We then waited in sadistic anticipation and we were not disappointed. We watched her face change from a delicate pink to an unhealthy purple and we were convinced there were tears in her eyes as she fled from the room. The alarm clock was never seen again, but we continued to taunt and tease her and quite regularly saw the various colour changes which never quite matched her vivid red hair.

I must just mention domestic science. I hated it and made the worst macaroni cheese ever. The room had high windows but by standing on the wooden lid of a flour bin, I could just see the boys playing football. That was much more interesting and I took my chance when the teacher momentarily left the room. Her return was rather earlier than expected and my descent very clumsy. There was a loud crack as the wooden lid split in two. I finished up knee-deep in flour with the room enveloped in a cloud of white dust. My embarrassment and humiliation were punishment enough. The wrath of the teacher was too much to bear and my dislike of cooking continues to this day.

2

Learning about Dates

Down the hill from our house, past the fish and chip shop and the bowling green, past row after row of identical terraced houses and my old junior school, and there it was! The house that was to become so familiar to me, the house where a young lad just 18 months older than me, lived with his parents and two older sisters. We had never met, didn't even know of each other's existence. Our paths had never crossed. He had gone to a different primary school and was now at a secondary modern school. His two sisters, one 14 years and one 12 years older than him, had not been allowed to go to the grammar school in spite of having passed the scholarship examinations. It was a waste of time for girls, so the parents thought. And as for the lad, he could forget any highfaluting ideas he might have about degrees and careers. The sooner he became a wage earner the better. He was an unplanned pregnancy, an 'afterthought' when both parents were well into their forties. He was a placid baby with three 'mothers' to look after him. Now he was older, he had adopted a quiet acceptance that his 'lot' was to leave school as soon as possible and start paying his way in life. Any ambitions he might have had were now just pipe dreams and quite out of his reach. His sisters had been working for a long time. Edith, the elder one, was a clerk at the Victory V factory and kept the family supplied with jelly babies and throat lozenges. Doreen had rebelled against working in a cotton mill – the fate of the majority of girls in this area of Lancashire. Instead, she had trained as a tailoress and was already very talented.

In my first years at grammar school, I knew nothing of the

interior of this house or of its occupants. The outside, however, was very familiar to me. It was a bigger house than ours but, like all the rest in the row, looked cold and uninviting. There was no garden to speak of – just a soot-black privet hedge behind a low stone wall and a pocket handkerchief 'plot' of rubble and weeds. The front door with its dark brown peeling paint was only a couple of strides from the street. The faded yellow curtains at the window were always drawn together. Marion, Jean and I often chose to walk home from school and our journey took us past this house. When pocket money allowed, we were drawn like a magnet to the most gorgeous confectioner's shop, just two doors away, with its irresistibly mouth-watering cakes and pies. Our usual purchase was a small bottle of lemonade for us to share and a bilberry pie each. To this day, I have never tasted better! None of the present-day plastic apology for fruit, but flavourful, real bilberries freshly gathered from the moors – delicious! These we would take to the house two doors away with its convenient wall for us to sit on and enjoy our feast. Then, grammar school girls or not, we would furtively dispose of the glass bottle and paper bags by pushing them between wall and hedge. This we had done for many months until the fateful day when the front door flew open and a large red-faced virago stood, hands on hips, swore abuse at us and threatened to have the law on us! Our punishment was to clear up all the mess, scrub the wall with soap and water and, whilst we were at it, remove all the weeds and tidy the garden. That was my first meeting with my future mother-in-law – she frightened me then and continued to do so until the day she died.

I suppose I must have been about 12 and had absolutely no interest in boys. Being in a co-educational establishment meant they were always there but, as far as I was concerned they could get lost. Then one day, halfway through the Latin lesson, I was handed a grubby scrap of paper with a scrawled, almost illegible message that read 'Meet you at the Saturday matinee. Frank.' He didn't need to specify where. The place for a first date was always the same. I could picture the hoarding – 'Queen's Cinema. 2 p.m. matinee. Every Saturday.'

I didn't fancy Frank but I did fancy going to the pictures, so with just a moment's hesitation, I scrawled 'OK' on the note and passed it back. That was on the Friday afternoon. It really was a last-minute invitation.

I didn't know what to expect. I had never done this before, but at least I thought he would be outside waiting for me. He wasn't. I messed around until nearly two o'clock and then thought Oh well, he hasn't turned up but now I'm here I'm jolly well not going to miss the film. I bought a ticket – the cheapest – and went in. I saw him straight away – in the back row with his blazer dumped on the next seat to 'save it'. He waved, moved his blazer and I joined him.

So I was expected to buy my own ticket, I thought. Perhaps that's another tradition.

'Hello,' he said. And then, after a long pause, 'You're late.'

'Um, yes – sorry.'

As I sat down, the lights dimmed and the trailer for next week began. I glanced at Frank in the dim light – what a twit! His face was all podgy and red, his hair looked as though it had never seen a comb. His nickname at school was 'Farmer' and I began to see why. His whole appearance reminded me of a scarecrow – an out-size one. His hands were enormous, all red and coarse. Definitely capable of heavy farm work. And his feet – they were huge, in their thick-soled clumsy boots.

He didn't speak again. Neither did I – there was nothing I wanted to say. I don't know what I expected to happen but, thank goodness, nothing did – until part way through the main film when I felt a hot, sweaty hand groping for mine. That was all. I allowed him to stick to my hand, thinking If he does anything else, I'll scream. It was horrible. I felt dirty just from his sticky heat.

At the end of the performance I couldn't get out of the cinema quickly enough.

Now he'll want to see me home, I thought.

He spoke. My goodness, it speaks, I thought.

He cleared his throat and then said, 'So long. See you on Monday,' and he was gone.

Monday morning I passed him a note which simply read 'I've chucked you.' He read it, scrumpled it up and never even looked at me. I had the distinct feeling he was just as relieved as I was.

After that first venture into the adolescent dating system, I became very wary of any further advances. I much preferred to keep my distance and I became a snob where going out with boys was concerned. There were one or two experimental dates but they didn't come up to expectations – or perhaps it was me! For whatever reason, they all shared the same fate.

I was therefore unprepared for the meeting that was to change my life. Gradually, I suppose, I had mellowed slightly in my opinion about boys. The biggest change had been in me joining the Tuesday night classes along with Mavis, Marian and Jean. It was at the Salem chapel in town and it was a course of ballroom dancing. It was great fun. I enjoyed being taught how to dance properly – the waltz and the foxtrot, the quickstep with lots of variations, the tango and rumba, fun dances like the valeta, conga and military two-step. It was an occasion for dressing up – short full-skirted dresses with shiny four-inch-wide belts, done up as tightly as possible to show off our tiny waists. We tottered around in uncomfortable high-heeled shoes with peep-toes and sling-backs. We had taken time and trouble over our hair – sleek 'rolls' held in place by carefully hidden hairgrips. Our faces had just a hint of decadence with touches of rouge, mascara, lipstick and powder – and, to add the final touch was the perfume, the cheapest from Woolworth's. Without it our image would not have been complete.

I felt pleased by the effort the boys had made. Shiny faces that really had been scrubbed clean. Sleek Brylcreem hairstyles, shirts with a proper collar and tie – and the pullovers, sleeveless Fair Isle affairs lovingly knitted by their mums.

Yes, I was definitely mellowing towards them!

The culmination of all this initiation into the world of dancing was to do it 'for real' at the weekend visit to the Imperial Ballroom. There was nowhere else quite like it. Everybody went there. Sometimes there were special appearances of the big bands. My favourite was The Squadronnaires – they were terrific. We danced to the most marvellous music. Famous names slipped easily off the tongue – tunes written by Glen Miller, Artie Shaw, Woody Herman and Duke Ellington. We danced to *String of Pearls, Woodchopper's Ball, Take the A-Train, Moonlight Serenade, In the mood, Perfidia, Pennsylvania Six-Five-*

Thousand, Begin the Beguine – and so many more. It was wonderful!

It was here on one of the special 'Big Band Night' affairs that I met Stan. I had noticed him on other evenings and thought he looked rather dishy. But this evening he asked me for a dance. It was immediately obvious that he had two left feet. He apologised for his lack of expertise, but it really didn't matter. He was such a gentleman compared to some of the other partners. The dance ended and he thanked me and walked away.

The rest of the evening passed in a haze. Then came the last waltz. He was by my side again and I joined him on the dance floor.

'I know we've only just met,' he said, 'but will you allow me to walk you home?'

I don't know what my reply was – but, whatever the words, the meaning was clear. 'Yes please.'

Then came the strangest few minutes of my life. I told the girls – they giggled and said, 'OK. See you on Monday. Don't do anything we wouldn't do!'

I looked round for Stan. He wasn't there. People were leaving – in groups, in twos – I watched and waited. After what seemed an eternity, he was back by my side, looking all hot and flustered. 'Sorry about that,' was all he said. 'I'll explain later.'

I discovered that he lived at the house with 'our' wall and that, horror of horrors, I had already met his mother! In spite of that, our friendship blossomed until soon we were seeing each other on a regular basis. It was months later when he confessed, 'Sorry about messing you about that first evening. I had to take Moira home first. We had decided that everything was finished between us but I had to make sure she got home safely – I'd promised her that I would.'

3

A Casualty of War

By the time I was 14 I had matriculated. I had passed all my school certificate subjects and I started working for my higher school certificate. But suddenly my whole world was turned upside down.

It was Dad who was the cause of all our worry. His problem had really started three years earlier when I was still only 11. It was the start of the Second World War that had sparked it all off. I couldn't understand why he was so badly affected by it. To me it simply meant the inconvenience of carting my gas mask around everywhere. The whole school had had great fun decorating the cardboard cases that we carried them around in, taking great pride in the unique designs that we had created. But we hated gas mask drill. Horrible smelly things they were. On the other hand, air raid drill was fun. It meant an escape from lessons and we very often chose not to hear the 'all clear' and stayed in the shelters until a search party was sent for us.

The other memories I have of the war were things like the 'Dig for Victory' campaign when parts of the school playing fields were converted to growing vegetables. Then there was the blackout. We had two-inch strips of sticky paper criss-crossing all the windows, which was meant to prevent broken glass flying everywhere. And the curtains were horrible black things to prevent any chinks of light from spreading outside. In our school, we also had a 'Save Paper' campaign. Only essential notes and exercises went into our 'best' books. All rough drafts and notes had to be done on Victorian slates with scratchy slate pencils. Sufficient slates and pencils appeared as if by magic from lofts and forgotten stores.

So that was my war. But how different it was for Dad. He had had a dreadful time in the First World War and had been suffering the consequences ever since. He would never talk about those awful days and I can only imagine what it must have been like. Once or twice, he would just mention the terrible hunger and thirst which was so great that they had to eat dry biscuits and 'bully-beef' crawling with maggots. There was no alternative and they would wait until it was dark so that they couldn't see what they were eating. Often the water would be straight from the river, filthy and germ-ridden. I am convinced that the duodenal ulcers that had almost cost him his life and had led to a lifetime of discomfort and pain were a direct result of those conditions.

Now, they had returned again, with a vengeance. He couldn't eat or sleep and was in constant pain. Nothing seemed to give him any relief and the local doctors all agreed that another operation would be dangerous and futile. They were powerless to help.

His time off work was a disaster. He was a 'tackler' at the mill, totally responsible for the smooth running of the looms. The weavers' wages depended on him. To have looms stopped for repair meant loss of wages for them. Dad, always conscientious, was now finding the sheer weight and awkwardness of the work too much for him. There was no regular money coming into the house, so Mum, who had 'retired' as a weaver at the same mill, got herself a job as a dinner lady at my former junior school. What with that, plus looking after Dad and dealing with all the household tasks, everything was taking its toll. She was tired and becoming increasingly worried and tearful. At the age of 14, for the first time in my life, I was suddenly aware of our circumstances. We were working class, we were poor and we were struggling. I began to feel guilty about enjoying life at school and even more guilty about looking ahead to the time when exams were behind me and I could go to university.

At the age of 14 I suddenly grew up. Subsidiary certificate at 15, higher at 16 – and then what? A couple of years' wait and three years at university? It was suddenly developing into a nightmare! Why had I been pushed through school so quickly? What good was it? I couldn't see beyond the hard facts that Dad was very ill, Mum was very worried and I must stop all my selfish thoughts about degrees and a career in teaching.

In desperation, Mum eventually sought out a specialist at Leeds General Hospital. I had no idea where she had got his name from, but what I did know was that it was a last resort. With an operation, Dad's chances of survival were slim. Without it, he would die. The specialist was prepared to try. His fees were very high and there would be extras to pay for. The total cost was probably a fortune for people in our circumstances. But Mum was adamant.

'Please try. I want you to try. I'll get the money somehow.'

And so it was arranged. The money was eventually loaned to us from Great-Great-Uncle Tom. It was all properly sorted out in a very businesslike way. Repaying the loan, plus interest, took years and years.

The next few months were so frightening. My whole world was falling apart. I suppose I had been so cosseted and protected that I had lived my life in blissful ignorance. The only blip had been my removal from junior school too early. But I was now revelling in the challenges and opportunities that were there for the taking.

That is, until now. Even to contemplate further education was selfish of me.

Within days of the decision to operate, Dad was taken to Leeds and the long agonising days of waiting began.

'I wish we lived nearer.' I heard Mum repeating those same words over and over again. Nowadays, from Nelson to Leeds is simple. But this was wartime, with a badly operating bus service and very few trains. Leeds could have been at the other end of the country. It was a journey fraught with problems.

The day of the operation arrived. I wasn't allowed to stay away from school but, I can tell you, not much school work was done that day. It seemed ages before any message arrived. But after the umpteenth phone call from the public call box, Mum finally got the message she had waited all day to hear. Dad had survived the operation! He was on the critical list and the success or otherwise of the operation was still unknown. We could ring, but no visitors would be allowed for several days.

I remember it was Saturday when we first visited him. The

17

journey seemed to take forever. We travelled by train, which was late, and we shared the compartment with two elderly ladies who never exchanged any words between one another. I don't think there was much conversation between us either. We were both of us deep in our own thoughts.

What would we find when we arrived at the hospital? How would he be? Was the operation a success? Would he be able to speak to us?

I had never set foot in a hospital before. I had never seen Mum look so worried.

If the journey was bad enough then the arrival in Leeds was much worse. The two elderly ladies were met by an even more elderly gentleman.

'Are you all right?' he fussed. And then, without pausing for a reply, he added, 'I wondered if you would make it. It was the worst air raid yet. There's been a lot of damage. The hospital got the worst of it.'

I thought Mum was going to keel over. Her face was completely drained of any colour. She looked at me with eyes that spoke volumes and whispered 'Come on ... he'll be waiting for us ... come on, hurry.'

As we turned the corner, we saw it. The hospital was still there! If there had been damage it wasn't immediately visible. Mum's hand tightened around mine – 'He'll be all right, you'll see.'

We were taken to a small single bedroom. 'Just a few minutes,' the nurse said. Within seconds my eyes had taken in the basic details – the small, high window with blackout shutters, the washbasin, oxygen cylinders, bottles and drips, the clutter of more bottles and dishes on the bedside table, the tiny bed with a mass of pillows – and Dad!

He looked to have shrunk. He was an awful colour, but it was Dad. He was alive and he even managed half a smile.

Gradually, the story came out. 'There was an air raid last night. They were moving everyone into the basement. But not me. I told them to leave me. I couldn't face being moved.'

His eyes closed. The effort of speaking, the memories of the previous night, his pain and his discomfort had exhausted him.

'He's going to be fine,' Mum said.

Dad's eyes opened momentarily. 'I'm all right,' was all he said. We left quietly.

4

Working and Walking Out

Dad continued to make progress. It was painfully slow and he had to stick to a very strict diet which he hated. He still looked far from well and I knew it would be a very long time before he would be able to work again. I secretly thought his working days were over.

My worry about going to university continued. I was now 15, and had taken four subjects at subsidiary level and passed them all. Mum had continued to voice her fears about the future and I had decided the best way forward would be for me to leave school as soon as possible. I had managed to convince myself that I didn't really want to go to university at all.

The day of reckoning had arrived. As with everything in my life, it was badly timed. It was too early for me to leave school without special permission and it was too late for me to change my mind. A meeting had been arranged between the headmaster, Mum and myself. In spite of my decision to leave school as soon as I could, there was still a little voice inside me telling me that further education was the best option. But it was wartime, the headmaster had many other more pressing and weighty problems and the little voice went unheard.

He listened sympathetically to Mum's account and then, all too easily and quickly, the decision was made. As soon as I had found employment I had his blessing to leave, with all his good wishes for the future.

I didn't know whether to laugh or cry, and one look at Mum's face told me that she had the same misgivings. There was relief but it was tinged with so much sadness.

And so my fate was sealed. My very first interview was also my last. The job was mine. I could start immediately as a very junior clerk in the Union Bank of Manchester (now Barclays) in Burnley. In November 1943 my working life began. I well remember my first day and the first question I was asked.

'Do you know what a cheque is?'

I had absolutely no idea. My knowledge of banking was zero. So I very simply had to start at the bottom. I took to the job like a duck to water and the grounding was very thorough. Very quickly I was as knowledgeable as the rest and I was given the opportunity to have experience of every department, all of which has stood me in good stead all through my life.

I enjoyed working as a cashier and meeting the customers. I enjoyed the local clearing of cheques, which gave me the chance to socialise with staff from all the other banks in the area. I revelled in the accounting. Our one bit of 'modern' equipment was a primitive adding machine, which I despised – it was much quicker to add up a column of figures in one's head. We sat on high stools, like something out of a Dickens novel, updating the enormous ledgers by hand. Daily interest rates had to be calculated, overdraft charges checked and, although the bank closed at 3 p.m., the staff were not allowed to leave until everything had balanced. One penny over or too little and everything had to be checked and re-checked until it was found. On a good day, we could be on our way home at 3.15. On a bad day, it could be as late as 6 o'clock before we got away.

After a couple of years' experience and well on the way to passing all the banking examinations, I became a 'relief staff member'. This meant that I could be sent to other branches in the vicinity if staff levels were too low because of holidays or illness. I enjoyed the work enormously and worked for a time at many local branches – Nelson, Colne, Bacup, Rawtenstall, Todmorden – and many others.

I continued to see Stan, often at lunchtimes. He was, by this time, working just over the road from the Burnley office at the Borough Building Society. He, too, was having experience in all aspects of building society work. He was only 'temporary'. The permanent staff would return when the war ended and he would have to finish. It was a big disappointment in his life when he was turned down for the forces on medical grounds. It was discovered that he had a damaged heart valve – probably the result of having had rheumatic fever when he was 13. It has never caused him any problems and he has always been accepted on any insurance policy. But the forces didn't want to know.

As well as seeing him at lunchtimes, we also met as often as possible after work. During the summer, that meant an evening walk. We both of us loved the countryside and there was no shortage of that around Nelson. One of our favourite walks was to Catlow Bottoms. We would make our way past all the posh houses in Halifax Road and over the stile on the left. The views were superb. We were high up and could look down to Walverden and all the rolling countryside around Catlow and up to Walton Spire. Topping them all was Bouldsworth Hill. The path led through meadow land and an old farm track to Hill Lane. To the next stile was by way of a cinder track and some uneven flags (paving stones to the foreigners). Then it was on to Robin Cottages and, after another couple of fields, Burwains House – a lovely old place, distinctly Catholic, with its own chapel, an exceptionally fine porch, stone plaques, coats of arms and an air of mystery, indicative of past strife, religious fervour, superstition and war. The next stile had five steps – we knew because we always counted them – then we had a choice, a pretty path on the left down to a wooded clough, or a path on the right which also led to the clough but passed Ecroyd farm. This was a Quaker homestead with a secret upstairs room which was always locked and a deep, dark cellar. It was a beautiful place with mellowed stone and a slate roof, bronzed with 300 years of ageing.

The clough was so pretty with its crystal-clear stream and carpets of flowers under the canopy of trees. This, to us, was Catlow Bottoms – but officially the name belonged to the farm house a little further along. The farm was a place for children with swings, see-saws, a stream for paddling and a place for picnics. We would linger by the old one-arch bridge over the stream and the ford in the road where the water slops over. We would stay by the side stream where it crossed the lane and dropped by four feet to meet the main stream near the slab bridge. It was a magical place, a place for making plans for a future together – a place for us to daydream.

Soon after we started going out together, I took Stan home and introduced him to Mum and Dad. He loved to come to our house, thoroughly enjoying the company, the warmth and especially the food, over which he went into raptures.

I didn't really understand why he was so fond of coming into our house until the day he plucked up the courage to take me to his house. At long last, I was going into the house with 'our picnic wall' and going to meet his mum and dad. I just hoped his mum wouldn't recognise me!

As soon as I entered the house I knew why he had been so reluctant. It was a cold, unfriendly place. A sad house in which its occupants existed in silent isolation. A place in which to eat and sleep but very little else.

Through the front door with its peeling brown paint was a dark passage, with more brown paint, peeling wallpaper and a floor covered with badly worn and faded linoleum. The passage led past the front room to the living room and the scullery. There was a pervading smell of damp. It felt cold, even in summer. It was a sad, unwelcoming place – never could it be called 'home'.

The door to the front room was always closed. The curtains at the window were always drawn. Many front rooms were only used on special occasions and at all other times kept behind closed doors with the furniture under dust sheets. But this front room was different. It was unused because there was nothing in there to use. No 'best' things, just a clutter of bits and pieces stowed away in cardboard boxes, piles of old newspapers, bits of leftover wallpaper and other items that 'might come in useful, one day'. It was cold and damp, and had that awful musty smell that I always associated with such places. It was horrible.

The living room was not much warmer. The fire never had enough coal on to give out much heat. There was a coal scuttle filled with coal but Stan's dad almost had to ask for permission to use some of it – and as for poking the fire to create a blaze, that was completely taboo. The room was spartan. The largest piece of furniture was a very old sideboard with a couple of photographs in cheap frames and a vase that I never saw with any flowers in it.

23

There was a large deal table, usually covered with a green woollen cloth. Stan's mum and dad occupied the two fireside chairs and, apart from some stand chairs, the only other furniture was a small cabinet on which was their pride and joy – a wireless!

Even in summer, Stan's mum and dad would be wearing thick jumpers. In winter, they would add an extra jumper, shawls or scarves and even mittens.

The window looked out onto the backyard – a desolate place, reached by five steep steps from the kitchen and surrounded by a high wall which prevented any sunlight from finding its way in.

The kitchen was squalid. There was a stone floor covered with bits of rush matting and rag rugs. There was an old wash-boiler and a mangle, an ancient gas stove with an assortment of iron pans and chipped enamel bowls. A couple of shelves were piled high with more pans, dishes and an assortment of plates and cups. The window was tiny, with frosted glass always wet with condensation. Patches of mould and mildew were clearly visible in many places.

That was downstairs. I was never allowed upstairs, so I can only guess what that was like. The house wasn't theirs. They paid rent to a landlord who had no intention of improving it in any way. Stan's mum and dad had never owned their own home and this was the third rented property in the town that they had lived in. His father had had a variety of jobs including that of pawnbroker's clerk – quite a lucrative trade in that area of Lancashire. He had then tried to run his own business as a gent's outfitter – but that was during the depression and, not surprisingly, never got off the ground. His last job was as a clerk in the Labour Exchange – again I expect he would always be busy.

Later on, when I was invited for a meal, I realised why Stan enjoyed eating at our house so much. My first meal at his house was a tiny fillet of plaice poached in milk and served on a completely white plate, with white sauce and a mound of white mashed potatoes. Out of politeness, I pretended to enjoy it, and thereafter was served with an identical meal every time I went. Later on, when I confided to Frank (Stan's brother-in-law) he laughed and said that he had had the same experience. His first meal there was tripe. Every meal from then on was also tripe. He didn't even like it – he was just being polite.

5

Music and Marriage

As well as the banking exams, I was also studying hard for my music diploma. I had started piano lessons when I was quite young – about seven years old, I think. Right from the start, it was a bit of a hit-and-miss affair. We had a real 'honky-tonk' piano, never in tune and with half its keys sticking. My teacher was Uncle Tom – the same uncle who came to Mum's rescue and loaned her the money for Dad's operation. He was quite deaf, so he watched rather than listened. He armed himself with a thick, black ebony stick which he would bring down smartly across my knuckles when he detected a wrong note. It certainly made me conscientious about practising – I was too afraid to do anything else. But he wasn't able to teach me very much. His own musical ability was very limited and I made little progress.

A combination of increased school work and decreased enthusiasm for the piano soon meant that piano lessons were put on hold. After quite a long gap, it was decided that I should have proper lessons with a qualified teacher. Mr Heaton was a wonderful teacher, very kind and very patient. He had been told that I could already play the piano a little bit, so I was asked to take along one of my pieces. I chose Elgar's *Chanson du matin*, quite confident that I could cope.

I couldn't! The right hand wasn't too bad – but Uncle Tom had never bothered about what was happening with my left hand, so it came as quite a shock to discover I had to use that hand as well.

Chanson du matin was my starting point with proper lessons which continued until I was ready to take some of the exams.

25

Lessons and exams went on until by early 1943 I had taken all the exams of the Trinity College of Music, culminating with the Advanced Senior Grade. I then embarked on a concentrated course of study as I worked for my diploma.

By this time I was working in the bank and was encouraged to continue my music by one of the other girls working there. Mary was a very keen pianist and we would compare notes about what we were doing. I went to hear her play at a local concert and she was very good indeed. We talked non-stop about music, even inventing our own musical code, using it to pass on messages. For example, humming a few bars of Ravel's *Pavan for a dead infanta* meant 'I need the toilet'. (Pav., short for Pavan, is also short for pay a visit.)

I was 18 when I took my diploma examination. I had to travel to Manchester and was glad of Mum's company. As usual, we were early. Mum always allowed twice as much time as necessary. I thought it would allow me time to sit down quietly and calm down. But it didn't work like that. As soon as we entered the waiting room, an official welcomed us and then said 'Ah, you are the diploma candidate. We don't want to keep you waiting. Would you like to go straight in?'

Francesco Ticciati, D.Mus.(Lond.), FLCM, introduced himself. His face was kind but inscrutable. I had no clue about what he was thinking. I went through the motions like an automaton – the oral tests, the sound tests, the scales and arpeggios, the sight reading and finally the examination pieces themselves. First Beethoven's *Sonata in D major, Opus 10 No. 3* and then Chopin's *Study No. 1 in G flat*. This is known as 'the black key study'. It is played almost entirely on the black keys and I found it horrendously difficult. It is very fast (*Vivace Brilliante*) but needs to be played with total clarity and precision. Both pieces sounded wonderful on the Steinway grand piano – how different to our apology for a piano at home. I felt pleased with my effort and hoped the examiner had been satisfied. I then had to answer questions about the pieces I had just played until, finally, the examiner stood up, extended his hand and I was dismissed.

It was several weeks before the official result arrived. Mum's face was beaming as she handed me the envelope. I looked at it –

26

and I knew! It was addressed to Miss Audrey Ellis, ALCM – I'd done it! I was now an Associate of the London College of Music – I had my music degree and the right to wear their cap and gown (which I never did because we couldn't afford to buy it).

Music was my main form of relaxation. Years later it was also the 'open sesame' to the fulfilment of one of my ambitions – long overdue – but at the age of 43, I finally gained employment as a fully qualified teacher.

On reflection, once I had decided to leave school and start work, the remainder of my teenage years were very happy. Stan and I continued to see each other and spent long hours roaming the countryside. We often made up a foursome with Enid and Harry, who soon became firm friends – a friendship that has grown with the years and still endures today. Enid had also attended the grammar school, although I didn't know her then. Harry's family had been close neighbours of Stan when they were both young lads. We all enjoyed the same things and weekends would find us out walking – perhaps around Pendle – to Roughlee, Barley, Newchurch or Fence, or further over still to Downham. Sometimes we would go in the direction of Clitheroe and Whalley and we would explore the places around there. At other times, we would catch a bus or a train to Skipton and then go walking in Wharfedale, which was so beautiful.

We joined the Ramblers Association and the YHA and were then able to have weekends away, staying overnight in the Dales or the Lake District. Our annual holidays would be longer breaks in the Lake District, North Wales or Scotland, again staying in youth hostels. We also went on organised holidays with the Holiday Fellowship where we explored Devon, Dorset and Cornwall. They were wonderful times.

On my twentieth birthday Stan and I got engaged. And on the third of June 1950, when I was 22, we were married.

Although the war had been over for several years, we were still recovering from the consequences of those times. Food was still rationed and coupons were needed to buy clothing. The only new furniture available was 'Utility'. I used some of my precious clothing coupons for a wedding dress and a dress and coat for going away on our honeymoon. Stan's sister Doreen lent me her veil and I wore it with an orange-blossom headdress. Harry was very smart as our best man and Enid and my cousin Sheila were bridesmaids. They made their own dresses and carried small posies of anemones, with some of the same flowers in their hair. Stan wore his first new suit for many years and looked extremely smart.

The reception was at a local café. It was a spartan affair of ham and salad followed by trifle and wedding cake. After the reception, we left for a honeymoon in Torquay. We were so happy and after a wonderful week returned to Nelson to start married life in our very own house. We had been saving for the deposit for a very long time and between us had managed to save £60. The house had cost us £600 and it was a dump. It was a tiny little terraced house in a run-down area of Nelson.

But we were blissfully unaware of all its shortcomings. We had been lucky with the mortgage, which had been arranged on special terms because of Stan's employment at the building society. But we were unlucky with my job. The rule in 1950 was that no married women could be employed by the bank – so I had had to leave. I soon found another job in a mill office but I didn't like it very much.

Between us, we worked on the house, ripping out cupboards and fireplaces and stripping paintwork and wallpaper. Gradually it was transformed – it was our 'palace'. My boss, the mill owner, gave us enough curtain fabric for all our windows. It had been part of an order for a customer and he had some left over. Stan's sister gave us her old electric cooker, which she had just replaced with a brand new one. A neighbour of Mum's gave us a table and four chairs – old, but still in good condition – and we treated ourselves to a Utility bedroom suite. We only had linoleum and rugs on the floor – carpets were well out of our reach. But we did have two comfortable fireside chairs.

We were so proud of our little home and saved hard to add to it. I hoped for a washing machine and perhaps even a fridge one day. But they were real luxuries that would have to wait.

Soon after our marriage, Enid and Harry got engaged and

within two years they were also married. Stan was best man and I was matron of honour. It was another happy occasion tinged with sadness as they had decided to move to Enid's aunt's house in Cambridge. Harry was a painter and decorator and hoped to start his own business. Chances of success in Nelson were limited but Cambridge was a much better bet. We visited them in Cambridge and saw them when they came over to Nelson. But, sadly, the weekend rambles by the four of us were now gone forever. Stan and I continued to walk but it was never quite the same.

We had been married for six years when our daughter was born. During my pregnancy Stan did something that was so typical of him and so endearing. He knew I was worried about living at the other end of town to my parents and he came home one day with sale particulars of a semi-detached house quite near them. 'Do you like it?' was all he said. I thought it was wonderful and told him so.

'That's good, then – because it's ours. I've put in an offer for it which has been accepted and I've sorted out the mortgage already.'

I was in a dream world – our little terraced house sold very quickly for almost twice what we had paid for it. And here we were in a three-bedroomed semi, reasonably close to both sets of parents and to Doreen. (By the way, his other sister, Edith, was miles away in Wimbledon which is why she doesn't get much of a mention.)

We had a bathroom and separate toilet, masses of cupboard space, a dining room and a lounge and a large kitchen. The garden was gorgeous – it had a greenhouse and, best of all, a view of Pendle Hill. The previous owners had left all the curtains – some of them lush velvet – and all the fitted carpets. I felt like a million-aire.

Anyway, here I was blissfully happy in our new surroundings and anticipating the imminent arrival of our baby. Just days before *the* date, we suddenly decided that the only thing wrong with the house was the hall and staircase. It needed brightening up with a lick of paint and some new wallpaper. So, nothing daunted, we arranged for the decorators to move in. We would normally tackle any jobs ourselves, but not this one. Stan was put off by the high ceilings, the mass of wood panelling that needed special treatment and the ten doors! And I was obviously not much use.

It was on their second day that I began to feel uncomfortable and wondered if things were beginning to happen. I was willing the workmen to leave early and hoping against hope that Stan would soon be home. My relief when I heard the front door open was tremendous. We rang the maternity home. They thought it was probably a false alarm and then added 'Come in, if you feel worried. There's no rush – first babies always take their time.'

A couple of hours later, we were on our way to the home. This was no false alarm, our baby was definitely on its way. She arrived in the early hours of the morning and I thought of Stan, all on his own. I imagined him pacing up and down, worried and unable to rest.

He came to see us on his way to work. He was over the moon.

'Poor darling, what sort of a night did you have?' I was all concerned for him.

'Smashing! Best night's sleep I've had for ages!'

I could have smothered him!!

I thought, for once in my life, I had timed things perfectly. It was usual to spend ten days in the maternity home, by which time I would have a beautiful hall and staircase and the workmen would be gone, taking all their clutter with them. Just right!

How wrong could I be? When Gillian was just three days old, one of the new mums developed a very high temperature and was very unwell. The doctor was called and then announced that it was scarlet fever – a notifiable disease that threw the place in a panic. There was nothing else for it. It had to be closed and all the occupants sent home, and then it could be fumigated. Without ceremony, the following day all mothers, expectant mothers and babies were sent home. Instead of ten lovely days of rest followed by a wonderful homecoming, we arrived to find the place full of clutter. Everywhere I looked, the only things I could see were tins of paint, paper, paste, brushes, pasteboard, ladders, dust sheets and workmen!

But they were wonderful days. Gillian was an adorable baby and grew into a real charmer. My mum and dad spent as much time as they could in our company, always ready to help out in any

30

way they could. Stan's parents were not quite so forthcoming. In their own way, they were very fond of her, but made it quite clear that they would never interfere unless we specifically asked them to do so.

Meanwhile, Stan was beginning to get itchy feet. The next chapter in our lives would very soon start to unfold.

6

The Move to Worcester

Stan had worked in every department of the building society. For quite a few years his employment had been with the Marsden Building Society in Nelson. The temporary job in Burnley had, as expected, come to an end when things started getting back to normal after the war. He was very happy with his work and, like me, had studied hard with all the necessary examinations. But he was beginning to feel very unsettled – he could see no possibility of further promotion unless he was prepared to move. He started to pore through the adverts in the *Building Society Gazette* and eventually saw one that caught his fancy and sent off an application.

Once again, quite unbelievably, timing played a crucial part in our destiny.

We had arranged a holiday in Southend-on-Sea, where Mum's sister, Aunty Amy, lived with Uncle Fred and my cousin Sheila. Gillian was just three and apart from a short holiday in St Anne's on Sea, had never really been to the seaside. We were travelling down there by train and it had all been carefully planned. On the very day that we had made plans to go, we were actually turning the corner of our avenue on our way to the station when I intercepted the postman, who had also just turned the corner.

'Anything for number six?' He handed me an envelope. It was addressed to Stan and it was a reply to his application. It was a request for him to attend an interview in Worcester. If we'd left home a minute earlier or if the postman had been a minute later we would have known nothing about the interview until our return from Southend, by which time it would have been too late. Who knows what a difference to our lives that would have made?

As it was, he had to travel from Southend to Worcester dressed in holiday flannels and open-necked shirt. There had been no time to go back and pack more suitable clothes. Fortunately, it apparently made no difference. He attended the interview and was offered the job.

Like so many more families, in order to prosper we had to be prepared to move. Our parents were very brave about it – they were pleased for us and didn't want to stand in our way. But what a sacrifice it must have been for them. Extended families, which had once been the norm, were becoming fewer as more and more people moved further afield.

Stan's new job was to start on the first of September 1959. He would be second in command in the head office of Worcester Building Society. The Secretary, Mr Barnes, spent a lot of time away at conferences and Building Society Association meetings, which meant that for a lot of the time Stan would take control. He would be in charge and would have to attend all the board meetings as part of his normal duties.

It was a frantic time preparing for the move. The house in Nelson had to be sold, the furniture put into store and temporary accommodation arranged until we had found a new place to live.

The building society in Worcester had sorted out rooms for us in Fernhill Heath, a couple of miles north of Worcester city. We had contacted the owner of the rooms to ask if there was anything we needed to bring. Once all our furniture and belongings had gone into storage, it would be too late. We were assured that all we needed would be provided – so we only needed clothing and personal bits and pieces.

The lady on the other end of the phone sounded very friendly and we both felt that we could relax a little bit.

The thirty-first of August 1959, the day before Stan's new job was to begin, is a day I would rather forget. I began to question the wisdom of leaving behind everything and everyone we knew and loved. With very heavy hearts, we said our goodbyes, promising everyone we would return to see them as often as possible. I couldn't look at Mum and Dad. It wouldn't have taken much for me to dig my heels in and refuse to go. They had decided against coming to the railway station with us, preferring instead to say their goodbyes at home.

As we turned the corner of their street I thought This is it! Whatever happens now is in the lap of the gods.

We were in the middle of a heatwave and we were overdressed for the weather. A trunk of clothing had been sent off in advance and we had packed as much as we could of what was left into our hand luggage. But we had to don the rest.

The journey was indescribable. Gillian was fractious because of the heat and neither Stan nor I had anything to say to each other. Eventually we arrived in Worcester and found the heat and the humidity overpowering. Shrub Hill Station is not exactly a place of beauty and the surrounding area is decidedly scruffy.

This was my first glimpse of Worcester and my heart sank. We got a taxi to Fernhill Heath. I tried to make myself feel more cheerful. At least Fernhill Heath looked a bit more presentable. But my depression continued.

The taxi pulled up outside the house and I was aware of someone peering through the curtains of the house next door. Just as nosey as anywhere else, I thought.

Eventually we were installed in our new surroundings. Miss Wiltshire was reasonably friendly. I decided she was perhaps a bit shy. We had been promised a double bedroom for ourselves plus the small bedroom for Gillian. The front room downstairs was also for us and we would share bathroom and kitchen.

It didn't work out quite like that!

'I'm sorry,' said Miss Wiltshire, 'You'll all have to sleep in the one bedroom. I'm using the small bedroom at the moment as the other is being decorated.' (Six months later we were still there and her bedroom was still being decorated!)

Downstairs, the 'all you need' that she had promised turned out to be a very small room with a wonky table and only two stand chairs. There was a sideboard with doors that stuck and one fireside chair. In the evenings when Stan was there, we had to take turns sitting in it.

The only heating was a coal fire which belched out thick smoke into the room if there was the slightest breeze. There was a two-inch gap between the bottom of the door and the floor. And the window, too, with its very flimsy curtains was a constant source of cold air and draughts.

In September, with the heatwave, those things didn't matter. But in the winter it was dreadful. It was then that I realised that Miss Wiltshire was using coal I had bought and taking provisions I had stacked in the larder and fridge which mysteriously disappeared before I had time to use them.

The 'curtain-mover' next door turned out to be a real life-saver. She was friendly and helpful and loved to have Gillian for a few hours to help. On baking day, the help was especially welcome as Gillian returned with home-made goodies that were very much appreciated. Another family over the road were also very friendly and they kept me supplied with home-grown vegetables and fruit.

Stan discovered the infrequent bus service into town was a nuisance and bought himself a moped. The job was working out well and I gradually relaxed and began to feel less homesick. With Stan at work the days were long and I spent a lot of time exploring the country lanes nearby – sometimes alone, sometimes with Gillian and at weekends with Stan too. There was also house-hunting! We tried to discover the best parts of Worcester but soon realised that everyone thought their house was in the best part. To us, Worcester was just a hotchpotch of good and bad all mixed together.

Stan's boss was having a house built just off the Bath Road in the south of the city. 'There's a bungalow being built just round the corner – why don't you go and have a look at it?'

Although we'd never even considered a bungalow, we thought we'd take his advice and just go and have a look. It was nice and we decided to go ahead with the purchase. It meant a longer stay in Fernhill Heath as we couldn't hurry the builders but eventually it was complete and at long last we once again had a home of our own.

It was March 1960 when we moved in. The furniture, reeking strongly of mothballs, came out of store. It was so nice to be reunited with it again. We found a lot of pleasure in sorting everything out and finding suitable spots for it all.

A new house meant beginning a garden from scratch. Mum and

Dad couldn't wait to come down and see where we were living. It was so lovely to see them and Dad was worth his weight in gold as he started clearing builder's rubble, digging and levelling. He had to be careful about doing too much but he was enjoying every minute. At last he was feeling useful again. But for the photographs we had taken of our 'wilderness' I would never believe what a mammoth task we had undertaken.

Looking at it now, the garden is so beautiful with its background of mature trees and shrubs. There is a paved area with seats, Cotswold stone retaining walls overflowing with aubretia in the spring. We have a secluded patio with specimen shrubs in special containers. There are so many bulbs in spring and bedding plants in summer and, of course, a large green lawn. There is more garden down each side with honeysuckle and roses, hydrangeas and cotoneaster, pyracantha and japonica – and yet another lawn at the front with more shrubs, heathers and an ever-changing border of flowering plants.

We both enjoyed gardening. It is relaxing for me, even now, but I'm afraid I have to have occasional help with some of the pruning and heavy work. The soil is heavy clay and very difficult to work.

7

One Birth and Several Deaths

When Gillian was seven and a half she was joined by a baby brother. Our family was now complete. We had always wanted another child but had begun to think it would never happen. This time, things were not quite so straightforward as when Gillian was born. For the first few months I was quite unwell. Not just morning sickness, although that was bad enough, but there were complications. To this day I don't know what was wrong but I was being very carefully monitored. Towards the end I developed toxaemia and was ordered to rest. If I didn't I was threatened with a long enforced stay in hospital. Mum, bless her, came down from Nelson and took over.

During the early hours of the twentieth of January 1964, I wakened Stan and he took me to the hospital. I was put into one of the wards and told to stay in bed and relax. That was the last thing I felt able to do. I was so uncomfortable and felt I would be far better if I could keep walking. When I couldn't stand it any longer, they relented and took me into the delivery room.

Breakfast-time came and went. I heard the clatter of crockery and squeaky trolley wheels but I was left alone. I couldn't have eaten anything but I was so thirsty. Then it was lunch—again I was missed out. I must have dozed fitfully during the afternoon. A young nurse poked her head round the door. 'Everything still OK?'

'Could I have a drink please?'

She disappeared and never returned. I was desperate.

At about 3 o'clock, I was suddenly surrounded by nurses and

was then surprised to see our own doctor. I still don't know why he was there.

His first words were, 'Get some liquid into her, she's dehydrated.' Then he was full of concern for me. Thank goodness, I thought.

Everything seemed to be happening at once and at long last our son was born. I still don't know for certain but I think that a Caesarian was what they had been contemplating.

Mum, anxiously waiting back at our house, was the first to hear the news. Just in time for her to tell Muriel, a dear friend and neighbour who had just set off to collect Gillian from school. She was delighted and of course she was able to spread the word to all the other mums waiting at the school. Then she told Gillian's teacher and, of course, Gillian herself. Never had news spread so quickly.

The next day Dad arrived in Worcester. There was no way he was going to be left out of the celebrations.

Our son, Richard, brought us so much joy. Gillian adored him and was proud to be his second 'mother'. Stan and I often looked back with nostalgia at all the happy times we had had. We had so much to be thankful for. We were so lucky. We still had both sets of parents and everything we could wish for here in Worcester.

The only real sadness had been Grandad. We were still living in Nelson and Gillian was about 17 months old. It was Christmas Day – the first Christmas that we had made such a fuss about because she had only been a tiny baby the previous year. We were in the middle of discovering that Father Christmas had been! He had eaten the mince pie that we had left for him – and drunk the glass of port – and he had left us some presents.

Gillian was so excited and we were just starting to open the parcels when the phone rang. It was Alan, my cousin.

'Oh hello,' I said. 'Merry Christmas.'

The voice at the other end sounded strange. 'I'm sorry.' he said. 'It's Grandad. We found him this morning. He died in his sleep.' Then there was silence.

I was too stunned to say anything and Alan was too upset. Gradually the information sank in – but it couldn't be true. Not Grandad. Grandad was an institution. He couldn't die – especially not on Christmas Day!

I'd never known my grandma. She had died when Mum was only ten years old. Grandad had done a wonderful job in raising the family – my mother, her three sisters and one brother (who was unfortunately killed in the First World War). Grandad had a hard life but he was always cheerful and jolly. I'd never known him to be ill. He loved to be out of doors looking after his allotment and his greenhouse. When he was 80, the local press had printed a full page article about him, using a special birthday photograph that Stan had taken.

Now, at the age of 84, he had slipped quietly away – just as he would have wished. Once we had recovered from the shock, we were just relieved that the end had been so peaceful.

Round about the same time, when Gillian was still only a baby, we had another awful experience. This time it was Stan's mum. I was still frightened of her – to me she was still a formidable lady – but nothing could have prepared us for the day she tried to commit suicide!

She had got up extremely early one morning and turned on the gas. She had sealed the gaps under the doors with towels and then put her head into the gas oven. What ever wakened Stan's dad and alerted him to the fact that something was wrong we'll never know – but he was just in time to save her. She was really serious in her attempt and she never ever forgave him!

In hindsight, I now know that she was very ill. She would talk to herself, repeating the same sentence over and over again.

'Oh, I do forget.'

The memory of those words now strikes a chill in my heart. I know for certain that she really did forget – she wasn't just putting on an act. I am now also certain that what she had was Alzheimer's disease! But when it all happened, I had never even heard the name. I don't think I could have ever got very fond of her but had I understood, there would have been compassion and help.

I have had to learn the hard way about Alzheimer's disease. It goes right back to when Stan's mother was staying with us – we were actually looking after her and I was becoming increasingly disturbed by her very strange behaviour. She would disappear out of the house and catch a bus to Worcester city centre. But, once there, she would not get off but would insist on being taken to Nelson! We had so much trouble about that until finally all the drivers knew about her and wouldn't allow her onto the buses. Every time she disappeared, I knew where to go looking for her. She would be sitting on the seat by the bus stop. Often, persuading her to come back to the house with me was extremely difficult.

Then I had trouble with getting her to wash properly. Having a bath became completely out of the question and she was quite sure her hair and her clothes never got dirty! I knew something was very wrong. I even used the word 'dementia' – but the word 'Alzheimer's' came very much later.

I need to go further back still to explain why she was living with us.

It was November 1962 – the thirteenth – when we had the phone call from Doreen. It was an urgent message asking us to get up to Nelson as quickly as possible. There had been a dreadful accident and Stan's dad was in Burnley General Hospital fighting for his life. He had been knocked down by a car just yards from his home. The driver had apparently been dazzled by the low winter sun as he turned the corner.

We now had our own car, thank goodness, so we wasted no time at all in leaving Worcester. But by the time we got to the hospital it was too late – Stan's father had died.

'The nurse said it was a blessing,' was all Stan could say. And then, much later, he added 'They wouldn't let me see him.'

We drove to my parents' house where we were able to stay until after the funeral. It soon became very obvious that Stan's mum was unable to do anything for herself. Doreen went to the house as often as she could but was appalled by its condition. It was only then that we realised how much Stan's dad had been doing and how well he had managed to hide from us just what he had had to cope with.

There was no way she could be allowed to stay there on her own. Arrangements were made for us to take turns in having her to live with us. Edith, in Wimbledon, agreed for her mum to go there first – for six months, we decided.

Then this timing business took over again. After only a couple of months in Wimbledon, everything was thrown into chaos again.

Alec (Edith's husband) died suddenly and very unexpectedly with a heart attack. Edith found it impossible to cope and so, long before we had expected her, Stan's mum came to Worcester.

That was early 1963. By early May, I had discovered that I was pregnant and was feeling so ill that Stan had a long conversation with Doreen and it was decided that poor Doreen would take over the reins again. Things deteriorated so quickly that very soon afterwards we all realised that the only solution was a place in a nursing home.

A few months later, Stan's mum died.

This chapter seems to have developed into an account of some very sad episodes in our lives. But they are the facts and I really didn't think they could be left out. They formed a very important part of our background. So, also, do the next two events, after which I promise to cheer up and think of happier times.

First there was Auntie Maggie. She was my father's sister – a spinster, very plain, very ordinary and very distant. I once wrote a poem about her which I entitled 'Grey'. It seemed to sum her up completely. She was a grey mysterious shape which never quite materialised. She was the second accident victim in our family. Again knocked down by a car, one very foggy evening – 'in the grey mist, when grey met grey'.

There couldn't be a third one? Surely not?

My cousin Alan had been more fortunate than me. He had been able to go to Manchester University, where he got his BSc Hons. degree. He lived in Stockport, where he was happily married with a wife, daughter and adopted son. He was a brilliant scientist with work taking him all over the globe. He and a colleague were travelling to a job contract in Gloucester when a large lorry crossed the central reservation of the M5 and ploughed straight into them. They were both killed instantly. They were not far from Worcester and the inquest had to be held here. The local newspapers printed the whole story, complete with graphic photographs. It was horrendous! Both Alan and I had been only children, but, brought up as we were only doors away from one another, attending the same schools and having the same grandad and aunties, we were more like brother and sister. I felt his loss tremendously. And the accident having happened so close to Worcester seemed to make it even worse.

That's the end of this sad chapter. I promise to make the next one much happier.

8

A Dream Fulfilled

Life in Worcester with our two children was rosy. There was never a dull moment. Mum and Dad came down and stayed with us whenever they could and we also made frequent visits up to Lancashire. Stan's sister and her husband Frank also visited us and we would take them to many places all around the area. We walked on the Malverns, Bredon, Clee Hill and we explored many lovely villages such as Cropthorne and Overbury. We discovered places with such lovely names – Wyre Piddle, Upton Snodsbury and the Lenches. Sometimes we would have a boat trip on the River Severn or walk along its banks past the cathedral, the county cricket ground and the racecourse. We would walk around the hop fields near home, or go a little further afield into the Cotswolds – Broadway, Stow-on-the-Wold, the Slaughters and Bourton-on-the-Water.

Sometimes, when Mum and Dad were here, they would babysit and Stan and I would take the opportunity to indulge in a bit of 'culture' at Stratford-upon-Avon – or perhaps an orchestral concert in Birmingham. Our local theatre, The Swan, was also a favourite place for an evening out.

Dad used to love a day's fishing and made good use of the Severn, which was within easy walking distance from our bungalow. His favourite spot was by the Ketch Inn, where he could also enjoy a refreshing pint. As Richard grew older, he also loved to 'help' his grandad – until he became the proud owner of his own fishing tackle and he would then go off on his bike to all his secret fishing spots on the Teme, the Lugg, the Wye or the Severn.

When Richard was about four and a half years old, it was my turn to get itchy feet. An idea was put into my head and, once there, it refused to go away. It happened when a neighbour told me that he was applying to Worcester College of Education to do a three-year teacher-training course as a mature student. Why had I never thought of that? All I'd ever really wanted to do was teach – and here I was with an excellent training college right on our doorstep!

Whatever could I be thinking of? I suppose I had already lost confidence in my abilities. I would never be accepted. But, even if I was, how on earth did I think I would be able to cope? Let's face it, the whole idea was impossible – just an idiotic pipe dream! For a start off, Richard wouldn't be able to go to school until the following January, long after the start of the academic year at the college. We hadn't a single relative living anywhere near and Gillian, bless her, although a very sensible and capable girl, was only just 12 – still only a child!

I tried to put the whole thing out of my mind and carry on as before. The trouble was that it just wouldn't stay forgotten. I spent the days daydreaming and imagining myself in front of a class of children. Always juniors, always round about the age of ten or eleven. I pictured their faces, eager to learn, bursting with enthusiasm and energy. I would be in the centre of it all, watching them, helping and guiding them forward in their pursuit of knowledge. Perhaps I would have to admit I was living in cloud-cuckoo-land and, in any case, the reality of teaching would be far removed from this dream. But dream it would have to remain. This time, my timing really was up the creek. Let's face it. I would never ever achieve my ambition. I would never become a teacher.

'What's the matter?' asked Mrs Percival. 'You're looking very worried about something.'

Mrs Percival was a lovely neighbour. She was Italian, born in Florence, and she had worked as as interpreter during the war. Now she was happily married to her wartime English sweetheart and lived close by with her three sons and one daughter.

'No, I'm not worried. Just a bit down in the dumps.'

Gradually, I found myself telling her about my impossible dream and pouring my heart out about how disappointed I was feeling.

'Oh, I can just imagine you as a teacher – you would be wonderful.'

And that was the end of the matter. Or so I thought! Imagine my surprise, therefore, when several days later she called me over to her house, full of excitement.

'We've been talking it over, my husband and I – and I can help out. Just you go and see the headmaster! I've a feeling he will be all in favour of you going to college and I'm sure he will agree to Richard starting school in September. Then there will be nothing to stop you.'

Her face was a picture. She was so enthusiastic and I found it was catching. But then, common sense took over.

'But wait a minute. Even if he can go to school, and even if I do get a place, what about things like late lectures, what if the children are ill, or you are ill – what then? There are bound to be all sorts of problems.'

'Nothing that we can't solve,' she said. 'I will collect Richard from school along with Wendy. I would just love to help. He can stay with us until you're home. Gillian, too, if you are worried about her.'

Her enthusiasm was infectious and very sincere. So much so, that I really did allow myself to get just a little bit optimistic about things. Not too much – I didn't want to raise my hopes only to have them dashed again. I talked it over with Stan and he agreed that it sounded like a very good idea.

'Don't forget,' he reminded me, 'even if there are late lectures, I'm home soon after five – so they aren't going to be too much of a problem. I know it's what you want – so go for it. I'm right behind you and I will help too. I'll help with everything.'

And so it was arranged. Mr Barnacoat, the Headmaster of Cherry Orchard School, agreed Richard could start a term early. Richard was thrilled to bits and was very keen. He had already been attending nursery school and was more than ready to start 'real' school. He was ready for the mental stimulation and the interaction with other children and adults that school would provide.

The only two hurdles now remaining were the application and the subsequent interview. There really was nothing to stop me. The first bit was easy. My application was acknowledged and an interview was arranged.

Then the doubts started all over again. I had opted for two of what I considered to be less academic subjects to study at main and subsidiary level. I would dearly have loved to take English and music but thought perhaps my brain power had diminished through lack of usage. I therefore chose needlecraft, which I adored as a hobby, and rural studies because of my love of gardening and the outdoors.

The day of the interview arrived. I had, as requested, taken along with me samples of my needlecraft. I was shown to a seat in the large entrance hall and instructed to wait until my name was called. It was then that I almost chickened out. A lady sitting next to me and just trying to be friendly completely demoralised me by asking 'Which one is your daughter?'

I very nearly turned tail and ran. I felt so humiliated. What on earth am I doing here? was all I could think.

The interviews – three, in all – actually went remarkably well. I was immediately put at ease by all the people I met. In fact, they were very encouraging and certainly didn't make me feel that I was too old. On the contrary, they put forward the very valid point that, unlike the majority who had no life experience other than school, I had far more to offer. This, they pointed out, was something often lacking amongst teachers of young children.

I was encouraged by this and thrilled to be told, before I left, that there was a place available for me provided all my home arrangements could be verified.

I was given a book list and, conscientious soul that I was, had devoured them all long before the start of the course.

Older than most I may be, I thought, but the grey cells are still intact and I will certainly put them to good use.

I was understandably apprehensive as I entered college on the first day. Everything had gone remarkably smoothly at home – the whole family, even Richard, supported me to the hilt. It was also the first day for my neighbour who had first planted the seed of an idea into my mind. Alf, too, was apprehensive. We had arranged to go together – safety in numbers, maybe.

My fears proved to be completely unfounded. I was never made to feel something of an oddity because of my age. I was immediately accepted by everyone – students, tutors, and all the members of staff. My confidence soared. This is going to be just great! I thought.

And so it proved to be. The three years simply sped by and I took it all in my stride. My family obliged by staying healthy all the time. Richard adored going to Mrs Percival's home. She was an absolute angel and did far more than I ever expected.

'I do it because I love him,' she would say to me, over and over again.

My college timetable was actually very kind to me. There were very few late lectures, so more often than not, I would be at home ready to greet the children, which was lovely for all of us.

I soon found that my education tutor expected me to put forward my more mature approach to many of the topics and, although it was quite daunting to begin with, the nods of approval all round soon gave me courage and I began to revel in my new role. The needlecraft course was wonderful. It was very much art-orientated, which suited me down to the ground. It also slotted in very nicely with rural studies, which took me out and about and opened my eyes even more to the wealth and beauty all around. In my mind, needlecraft and nature could never ever be separated again. I only had to look around and everything I needed was there. The shapes, the lines, the symmetry, the colours, the textures were all there and my designs just flowed. I still spend a lot of time creating embroideries from natural objects and experimenting with new techniques. There is never enough time in any one day to do everything I would like.

At the end of the three years my personal tutor sent for me.

'The examiner would like a few words with you.' And, on seeing my face, quickly added, 'Don't worry. He always chooses one or two people to interview. You've got nothing to fear.'

I walked out of the interview room in a pink haze. I had been told – 'unofficially, you understand' – that I had passed with flying colours. A few days later the official list was posted on the noticeboard. I couldn't believe my eyes – not only had I passed but I had gained distinctions in everything!

I'd done it! At last I had achieved my lifelong ambition! Now all I needed was a job.

My qualification came just when jobs were getting rather hard to come by. I also thought I was under the distinct disadvantage of lack of flexibility in where I could work. Any position would, of necessity, have to be in Worcester because of transport problems. Perhaps my age would also go against me. I began to get quite worried.

Thank goodness my worries were short-lived. I attended just the one interview and met John again. He had been a fellow student, very full of his own importance, which, quite frankly, only he believed in. He condescended to speak to me.

'They need someone for music. I can play the piano. I've been learning for six months, so I shall be all right.'

Oh, the cheek of him! How dare he profess to be a musician in such a short space of time! It was because of his absurd pronouncement that when I was asked about music, instead of my usual reticence, I spoke firmly and told them that I had all the right qualifications and I would be keen to develop music throughout the school.

That was it! The job was mine and I could start at the beginning of the school year.

We were on top of the world. Proud of our achievements, happy with our wonderful family, our prosperity and our lives so far removed from the harsh backgrounds of our childhood.

But we neither of us knew that the biggest storm cloud of all was threatening and would very soon be closing in on us.

PART TWO
THE STORM BEGINS

9

A Holiday That Wasn't

'Come on then, hurry up – it's time we weren't here!'

The irritation in my voice was very evident. This leaving for work at 7.30 every morning was beginning to get me down. In fact the whole of Stan's move from Worcester to the new head office in Wolverhampton was causing me a great deal of concern all round. I still didn't know exactly what was going on and any attempt by me to try to find out was met with a variety of replies leaving me more confused than ever.

'Don't worry yourself about me – I'm OK. I never know from one day to the next just what I will be doing. I just fit in wherever I'm needed.'

That didn't sound right to me. The building society was noted for its staff management. The recent expansion and amalgamation with other societies had meant many changes but all would have been very carefully worked out.

'What were you doing yesterday?'

'Oh, for goodness' sake stop pestering. Just leave me alone.'

Stan's pinched face and resigned expression said it all. He had been deeply upset by this move. He hated Wolverhampton. He resented the daily journey, the loss of job satisfaction, the place, the new members of staff – everything. But there was more to it than that. I couldn't put my finger on it but I was certain that something was very wrong.

It had become routine for Stan to drop me off at school on his way to Wolverhampton. I was there by eight o'clock. How ridiculous – the only other person on the premises was the caretaker!

But I tried to turn it to my advantage. My lessons were always carefully planned, my marking up to date and my classroom display well mounted and changed quite frequently. I had time to plan ahead, which also meant there was less lesson preparation to do at home. Even so, given the chance, I would still have preferred an extra half-hour in bed and a later departure from home.

Every day I was home long before Stan. Our evening meal was usually something light as we had both had a substantial meal at midday and the last thing I wanted to do after school was to start cooking.

But I had begun to have doubts about that. Whenever I asked, 'What did you have for lunch today?' I always got the same reply.

'I've forgotten.'

'You can't have.'

'Well I have. Just leave me alone.'

I was becoming increasingly worried. Stan was looking more and more haggard and withdrawn. Our neighbours were beginning to notice.

'Poor Stan. Wolverhampton is really getting him down,' said Peggy and Syd.

'Is Stan all right? He doesn't look at all well,' said Olive and Jim.

I continued to worry. He shut up like a clam whenever I mentioned work. He began to forget things and he lost things. He had to be reminded several times about things that should have been routine. 'Have you enough petrol in the car?' 'Don't forget to collect your suit from the dry cleaners.'

I didn't dare grumble about anything – that would only make matters worse. How I wished that he had never had to go to Wolverhampton.

Months went by. I had long ago stopped quizzing him about work. It only upset him. He went off to work each morning like some sort of robot programmed for the rest of the day.

At the end of May we decided to have a break. We would take the caravan to the site at Longleat, home of the Marquis of Bath. From there, we would rediscover some of our favourite haunts and explore new places. The preparation was all down to me. I didn't mind that but I was vaguely disconcerted about his indifference.

There was no checking to see if I had thought of everything, just an air of detachment about it all. Perhaps I had pushed him unwillingly into going away for a few days. Perhaps he would rather have relaxed at home. Perhaps ... oh, to hell with it ... we were jolly well going... We needed a break and it was time he pulled himself together!

The journey was uneventful. The caravan was pitched and I began to relax. We were in a delightful spot, the weather was perfect and we treated ourselves to a meal out followed by a long walk in the lovely Wiltshire countryside before returning to the caravan for the night.

Now that there were just the two of us, we had exchanged our family-sized caravan for a luxury two-berth model. The twin berths would easily convert to a double bed but, more often than not, we left them as they were – and so it was on this particular evening. I must have fallen asleep almost immediately, only to be awakened in the early hours of the morning by his restlessness. I could hear him tossing and turning. He was moaning quietly and sniffling ... surely he wasn't crying?

'What's the matter? Are you ill?'

'I'm all right. Don't worry about me.'

'Are you warm enough?'

'Yes.'

'Would you like me to make you a drink?'

'Oh, stop fussing. Just leave me alone.'

That was said with such vehemence, such finality, that I felt further questioning would be useless. I lay there quietly, listening to him. Eventually he became less restless and his heavy breathing finally convinced me that at long last he was asleep. Perhaps in the morning he would tell me what was wrong.

The morning dawned brightly and the sun had already made its appearance. It was going to be a beautiful day. Stan didn't mention anything about the previous night, so I left well alone.

We decided to spend the day in the gardens of Stourhead and found them just as wonderful as always. It was a warm spring day, warm enough to sit for a short time and enjoy the sunshine. I gradually relaxed. Whatever the problem had been during the night seemed to have completely disappeared. I had packed a picnic lunch and we sat surrounded by the glorious spring colours with their backdrop of blue sky and the rich reds of the magnificent acers. After lunch, we explored the village and the area all around, finally treating ourselves to a gorgeous afternoon tea.

That evening we were both exhausted. He was asleep before me. Thank goodness for that! I thought. I turned over and soon drifted off myself.

It must have been somewhere between three and four in the morning when I heard him. I listened quietly – he was awake – he was sniffing – he was quietly blowing his nose – he was sighing – he *was* crying! This time I knew.

'Stan.'

'What?'

'What's the matter? There's something wrong, I know there is. Whatever is it?'

His sobbing became uncontrollable. 'Oh dear, oh dear ... I'm sorry – so very sorry.'

I was out of my sleeping bag straight away and went and put my arms around him. He clung to me like a child. 'I'm so sorry, so sorry,' was all he could say.

'What is it – what's worrying you?'

There was a long pause and then – 'I'm going to have to tell you. I didn't want you to know but you'll have to.'

'Darling, what is it?'

'I'm ... I've been made redundant.'

It all came out in a rush. He was convulsed with further sobbing, then the whole story emerged. The previous day, on the very day we had started our break in Wiltshire and just ten days after he had celebrated his fifty-seventh birthday, he had been quietly told that his services were no longer required. He had been given three months' notice and on the thirty-first of August 1983 he would have to finish.

His story was mixed and very muddled. He was in a state of shock.

'I'm not the only one, you know. They've stopped lots of us.'

'Who else?'

'Oh, I don't know. I think it's just me – why me? Why have they picked me?'

'I thought you said there were other people.'

'Yes, there are. Well, perhaps there are. They wouldn't just pick me, would they? I haven't done anything wrong. I've always worked hard – I've always done my best. What are we going to do? I just wish I was dead.'

My mind was in a turmoil. It was obvious that I wasn't going to get much sense out of him. I wasn't going to find out the truth – at least not at this stage. My gut reaction was to get home. I wanted to be on familiar territory, somewhere safe, somewhere to gather my thoughts together. I needed to be able to give my whole attention to what was happening, somewhere where I could protect my darling husband, where I could take over and try to sort things out.

The full significance of what was happening suddenly hit me. His vagueness about his work in Wolverhampton, his forgetfulness, his indifference about everything – and now this! This wasn't just redundancy. This was much, much more! Something was horribly wrong – something that I had only just become aware of – and, even worse, something that I suspected Stan had not realised, and perhaps never would.

There was no more sleep for either of us. We sat in the half-light, warming our hands around mugs of hot tea, both of us deep in our own thoughts, neither of us saying anything.

In the cold light of dawn, I knew there was no point in staying on at Longleat. We packed the caravan, hitched it onto the car, settled our bill and left for home. On an impulse we stopped at the garden shop and treated ourselves to a glorious *Acer palmatum*. It was something we'd always promised ourselves but had never got around to buying. Now, 14 years later, it is so beautiful – especially in the spring – a bitter-sweet reminder of that day so many years ago when our lives were so irrevocably changed forever.

As we made our journey home we were both very quiet. Stan had withdrawn within himself again and I had a lot of thinking to do. One of us, at least, had to get some sort of normality back into our lives. I had no idea of what the future would be like but somehow we would cope. After all, Stan was not the first person to be made redundant – it was happening to lots of people all the time.

Our neighbours had been very surprised to see us home again so soon.

'Hello – what are you doing here?' And then, sensing from our expressions – 'Is everything all right?'

Before I could say a word, Stan had jumped in with both feet. 'There's nothing wrong. We're entitled to change our minds, aren't we?'

With that, he stormed into the house, leaving me open-mouthed and Olive and Jim stunned into an embarrassed silence.

'I'm sorry,' was all I managed and I too fled indoors. They were the nicest neighbours anyone could ever wish for. Kind and thoughtful, friendly and helpful – but never intrusive. Now, what must they think of us?

I would have to sort it out. I would have to tell them. After all, people would have to know soon. In three months' time there would be no job. But at this moment Stan was my first priority.

He had quietened down. He was sitting on the settee and staring into space, his face pale and drawn and looking suddenly old and vulnerable. I joined him and together we sat in silence. He needed time. He was not yet ready to accept all that was happening. He was not ready to talk.

Much more worrying was my realisation that he was ill. It wasn't just the shock of losing his job, it was something far more sinister than that. I blamed myself for not having seen the signs long before now.

I began to remember little details about previous years. For instance, there was that time in Lyme Regis when he got so angry about the difficulty he was having in putting a new film into his camera. Photography had been his lifelong interest. He did everything himself – developing, enlarging, printing. He had won prizes for his work, he had put on exhibitions – but now even the simplest thing had become too much for him to work out. I asked if I could help but was left in no doubt that any interference from me was quite unnecessary. He blamed the film, the camera, the light – anything and everything – but never himself. From that day in Lyme Regis his interest in photography had steadily declined. Instead of being worried, I think I had just felt relief that he was no longer carting all his gear with him everytime we went out.

56

Sitting there quietly, I too began to think. For two years, his unhappiness at having to go to Wolverhampton had worried me. But now I was very worried indeed. What if his inability to tell me what exactly he was doing there was because he couldn't remember? What if he was being made redundant because he was no longer coping? No – surely it couldn't be that. Not my intelligent, reliable, conscientious and hard-working husband. Of course it couldn't be that. After all, he wasn't the only one being made redundant. It was all the mergers and takeovers – it was just another staff-cutting exercise. That's why they had waited until his birthday – it made it easier to work out how many years were left until normal retirement age – that was it. But, wait a minute! Just who were the others? They couldn't all have birthdays in May! I remembered his vagueness when he told me, and the more I thought about it, the more certain I became that there were no others – just him – he was the only one!

Whatever were we going to do? Our world had suddenly crumbled and fallen apart. Thank goodness my job was still safe. Richard was only part way through his university course but nothing that happened to us was going to affect that. We would still manage. Then there were problems with my mother. She was still in Lancashire, still trying to lead an independent life – but advanced arthritis was rapidly taking over and I could see the time approaching when our entreaties to her to come and live with us were going to be accepted. But that was in the future. It was the present that was concerning me now.

I musn't let Stan have any inclination of how worried I was becoming. After all, it was only this job that was at stake. There would be plenty of others and it would be good for him to find something with a lot less responsibility. But first I must get him well again. I must make an appointment to see the doctor.

10

A Visit to the Doctor

It was a horrible time. At the start of the following week, Stan went off to Wolverhampton as usual. He was at the beginning of his three months' notice. He made no mention at all of what had happened. But for his haunted look and unnatural pallor (which I hoped was only obvious to me) everything was outwardly exactly the same.

I had been able to have a quiet word with Olive and Jim. They were shocked and very sympathetic.

'Not Stan – he's the last person to . . . oh, we just can't believe it. Why him? He does so much for them, he's so knowledgeable, so reliable . . . not Stan, it just can't be!'

I listened. I nodded. I pretended to agree. But my mind was already converting everything they said into the past tense. 'He used to do so much for them – he was once so very knowledge-able, he used to be reliable.'

For the umpteenth time I asked myself the same question. Why, oh why had I not seen the signs for myself?

My mind was made up and I made an appointment to see the doctor.

Doctor Roberts listened in silence as I explained what was happening and voiced my fears. He nodded but said nothing. I felt I had to say more. The words came tumbling out, jumbled and incoherent. I kept excusing myself, kept apologising for not making myself clear. What else could I say? Why didn't he tell me to stop worrying? Why didn't he say something? I began to wish I hadn't made the appointment. I felt that perhaps I was wasting his time.

Then he spoke. 'I'm sorry to hear this. It must be rather worrying for you.'

Rather worrying! I thought. Goodness me, what had to happen to make something really worrying? I wished even more that I hadn't come.

He continued. 'It sounds to me like pre-senile dementia.'

The words penetrated like steel. 'Pre-senile' – that's before one is old. And 'dementia' – that's madness, isn't it? Those were my thoughts but I couldn't find the voice to say anything. What I did manage was 'What can you do? What can I do?'

With the air of one who has said all there was to say on the subject and was already thinking of the next patient, he stood up, extending his hand, and simply said, 'Nothing. There's nothing that can be done. But don't worry, you'll cope.'

And that was it. My husband was losing his mind and there was nothing anyone could do about it.

I walked out of that surgery with the feeling that everything had suddenly come to an end. Like an automaton, I found my way to the bus and went home. I could hear the birds singing, I could see the flowers all bright and cheerful and the whole atmosphere full of laughter. How could everyone behave like this? Didn't they know how I was feeling?

I escaped into the quiet of the house, shut myself into the bedroom and allowed my feelings and all my pent-up emotions to take over.

The thirty-first of August 1983 – a date forever etched in my memory. This was it. This was the last time Stan would be going to Wolverhampton. He was so quiet, so resigned. I hadn't been able to get through to him. For the first time in our marriage I didn't know how he was feeling, I could only guess. There seemed to be a quiet acceptance, even relief about what was happening. But I also knew he didn't want me to worry and his attitude was probably a cover-up for my benefit. I had tried to talk to him, and tell him that nothing mattered any more, just as long as he was all right. He had nodded, given me a hug and simply said, as he had hundreds of times before, 'I'm OK.' And with that, I had to be satisfied.

I wondered what his last day would be like. A few days earlier, I had received a phone call from an unknown female voice.

'Hello, is that Mrs Brown? I work with your husband and a few of us would like to buy him a leaving present. Have you any idea what he would like?'

I found myself saying 'Cut glass. He loves anything in cut glass, he collects things like decanters.'

As I said it, I thought rather uncharitably of others who had left at the normal retirement time. There had been parties. They had been given a really good time and always a lovely gift. I had heard nothing about any party, but at least there would be a present. It was my fervent hope that they would be kind to him – that his last day would not be too traumatic. How I wished that I could have been there with him but, of course, that was unthinkable.

The new school year had not yet started so I was at home. I still had work to prepare but not today – I couldn't concentrate on school today. But there was no relaxation either. I had no idea when to expect him home but I wanted to make a special effort to have everywhere just as he liked to see it and some of his special favourites carefully prepared for his meal.

I listened for the back door to open – he always came in that way, it was nearest to the garage. Then I remembered – there might not be a car any more. He had had the option of buying it from the building society but he had not taken up the offer. Of all the company cars there had been, none had given more trouble than this one. There had been so many faults with it and it had been in and out of the garage like a yo-yo. We had therefore decided to go for a smaller, more economical and brand new car instead.

At last, I heard footsteps and in he came through the back door as usual. I could tell nothing from his face. It was expressionless. I took his briefcase from him and gave him an extra-special hug and kiss.

'Well, that's it. I've said goodbye to that place and I'm not sorry.'

'How was it?' I hardly dared to ask.

'Great!' (If only I could believe him!)

'How did you get home?'

60

'No problem. I used the car as far as Worcester, then I dumped it in their office car park and stuck the keys through their letter box. They can sort it out now. I've done with all that. Then I caught the bus.'

'Oh, darling . . . I'm so sorry . . . I wish . . .'

'Sorry! Sorry be blowed! I'm just glad it's all over. They can stick their job. I've finished with the lot of them. That's it – finished – *finito*!'

There was a long pause. I hadn't been sure of what to expect but certainly not this. There was real venom in his voice. Real anger. I had expected some show of emotion but anger was not one of the ones on my list.

Later that evening, after our meal, we were sat together in the lounge and he started to talk. Slowly and quietly at first but then the words came tumbling out and I began to get a real insight into what his last working day had really been like.

'I didn't get much work done today – but then I didn't really expect to. They kept coming, one or two at a time. Do you know, I've been there two years and I still don't know half of them. Not a bit like the Worcester office. They were a smashing lot.'

There was a long silence and then, 'I didn't know Frank Watson was retiring today.'

'Was he? I didn't realise he had reached retirement age.' I didn't really care about Frank Watson. He was one of the staff members who had arrived on the scene during one of the takeovers. I'd only met him on a couple of occasions and had found him loud, arrogant, full of his own superiority and determined to get to the top regardless of anyone else.

'I only found out today,' Stan continued. 'They asked me if I was going to his party.' His voice choked. 'How could I? I didn't know about it. Nobody told me he was finishing. I didn't have an invitation.' His voice faded away and I could see that he was near to tears.

So that was it! That was what was making him so uncharacteristically angry and upset.

'Oh, darling, darling, please don't get upset about him. He's not worth it. If he didn't even have the courtesy to invite you then he's sunk even lower in my estimation.'

61

I could have saved my breath. He gave no indication that he had heard me. 'Just imagine. He completely ignored me! Anyway, I didn't want to go to his stupid party ... so ... I (his voice choked again) ... when it was five o'clock, I just got my things together and left. I don't think anyone saw me go.'

There was another long pause and then – 'Oh, by the way, a few of the girls signed a card and gave me this. You can have a look at it if you want.'

Before I had time to reply, he stood up and walked off into the bedroom without even saying 'Goodnight.'

And that was it. It wasn't even nine o'clock. I looked at the small parcel he had handed me and read the card. I didn't know any of the names but I suppose I should have been feeling grateful to them. I finally opened the parcel – it would be a decanter. How wrong could I have been! The money collected had obviously not been sufficient for that. Instead it was a very small cut-glass jug and two whisky glasses. Not much for 23 years of dedicated service.

Months later I was told that as well as a party, Frank Watson had been presented with a complete tea service in the finest Worcester porcelain.

My eyes were swimming with tears as I pictured him in that vast alien place, full of strangers that he had never got to know and had never made him welcome. I pictured him alone, as he gathered together his bits and pieces and slipped quietly out of their lives. He was never one to make a fuss. To leave quietly was so typical of him. But what must he have felt like? What thoughts must have been going through his head? I wanted so much to find the right words of comfort, to hug him and hold him ... But not yet ... he needed to be quiet. He needed time to come to terms with what was happening. And I, too, needed time to think.

62

11

Mother Joins the Family

I seem to have spent an inordinately long time reaching this stage of my book. I suppose it's typical of me. Just like the title, 'a matter of timing' – I am procrastinating, reluctant to get to the real crunch and my real reason for putting pen to paper.

I suppose I could write a complete book about the fulfilment of my dreams and all the wonderfully happy times we had as a family, but I will limit myself to just a couple of paragraphs and then get down to the real nitty-gritty.

The children first. Gillian passed her eleven-plus and went to the grammar school for girls, where amongst other things she was taught the clarinet and I was able to accompany her on the piano when she took her exams. She then went on to study English at Lancaster University, where she was awarded a BA (Hons) degree and where she also met her 'Prince Charming', to whom she is now happily married, and lives in Berkshire with two gorgeous sons, Simon and Richard.

Our son, Richard followed in her footsteps, eleven-plus then Worcester Royal Grammar School, followed by a BSc (Hons) degree from Newcastle University. He is still 'thinking' about marriage but hasn't quite got round to it yet. He lives in Bedfordshire and commutes to London daily to his job as an environmental scientist.

As for me, I did get the first job I applied for with a graded post for music. I did teach ten- and eleven-year-olds and enjoyed every minute. I was able to combine my love of nature with my two other abiding passions – art and needlecraft. I was in charge of display in the school and also helped with school visits to Wales, France and Belgium. I also attended two in-service courses for teachers – Junior French '*Voix et Images*' and Junior Art – for which I gained a distinction and the highest marks in the county. For a time, I was acting Deputy Head whilst he was away on a year's training course. Not bad for a 'late-starter' – but just to get my head back to its normal size, then came the crunch, the agonising decision I had to make about finishing work in order to look after Stan.

So that's it. A précis of our family life.

Now for a bit more about my lack of timing ability.

I decided to retire in 1985. A decision which came about because of two very unfortunate events which happened after Stan had had to finish work. But first of all I must tell you that my father had finally succumbed to his lifelong battle against illness and had died at the age of 78, leaving Mum on her own. She was crippled with arthritis and we tried in vain to get her to come and live with us.

'Not whilst I'm able to manage' was always her reply. That was until 1984 when, after a series of falls necessitating stays in hospital, her doctor issued a final ultimatum – 'A nursing home or your daughter's'.

That was it. She would come to Worcester. All the arrangements went smoothly and I felt that it would work out well. There was nothing wrong with her memory and Stan was still able to do routine jobs around the house. Between them, they would manage. I would leave a midday meal for them and do the main chores myself when I came home from school.

It actually worked very well indeed and after she had been with us for several months, she wanted some of her personal possessions bringing down from Nelson. (Always the optimist, she still hadn't decided to put her house on the market as, when she was well enough, she would be able to go back home!)

We would have to make the journey there and back in one day and Olive and Jim very kindly promised to make sure Mum was all right whilst we were away.

This is when unfortunate event number one happened. We hurried through everything we had to do in Nelson. The car was

64

packed with the things Mum had asked for, we had eaten our picnic lunch and by mid-afternoon we were all ready to leave. But first, we must just call and see Doreen and Frank – just for a few minutes. They persuaded us to stay for tea. We checked on the phone with Olive and Jim, who assured us that all was well. Even so, I was slightly worried by this later than anticipated start to our journey home. I consoled myself with the fact that Mum was OK, that Stan had had a bit longer to rest and that we had both had sufficient to eat.

Halfway home, at one of the service stations, it was already dark when we pulled in for petrol. And then – horrors of horrors – Stan, instead, of paying, walked off into the darkness and disappeared.

He must have gone to the toilet, I thought. Why on earth didn't he go and pay for the petrol first?

Then I waited . . . and waited . . . and waited!

The two men in the office were watching me with suspicion and I began to get very worried.

Finally, I got out and said, 'I'm sorry. I don't know where he's gone and I can't pay you, I haven't enough cash on me.' That was perfectly true but I felt dreadful.

They muttered something unintelligible and I went back to the car. What on earth had happened? Where had he gone? I should be out there looking for him, but I daren't leave the car unlocked with all Mum's stuff in it. And if I locked it, I wouldn't be able to get back in again. What a mess. Whatever was he playing at?

After what seemed like an eternity, I suddenly saw him – out there in the gloom and completely lost. I got out of the car and shouted. Thank goodness he heard me and started walking towards me.

'Where have you been?' I yelled.

'I've only been to the toilet,' was his reply and then he added, 'What are you making such a fuss about?'

The bill was finally settled and we set off again. The two men stood outside and watched us until we were out of sight. I felt as wobbly as a jelly.

The second happening was whilst I was at school. I came home and as usual I went straight into the lounge to Mum. She looked so

65

distressed that I immediately said, 'Mum, what on earth's the matter?'

She burst into tears and said, 'I don't know what to do. Just take me to the toilet, quickly.'

I got her into the wheelchair and sorted her out.

'Where's Stan?' I asked. He had always been excellent at helping her when I wasn't there. Just as long as he was there to push the wheelchair she was then able to manage on her own.

'I don't know where he is. I haven't seen him all day – and I'm so hungry and thirsty.'

The tears started again and she was inconsolable. I discovered that the meal I had left for them was still untouched in the kitchen. I quickly made her a drink and gave her some food.

'Oh, Mum – I'm so sorry. Have you no idea where he might be? I'll have to go and look for him. Are you all right now? Are you comfortable again?'

'Don't worry about me. Just you go and find him. Oh dear, oh dear – I am such a nuisance, aren't I?'

'Of course you aren't a nuisance. It's my fault. I should be here all the time and then I could look after both of you.'

And that was when I decided the time had come for me to hand in my notice.

I soon found Stan. He was in the garage, arranging plant pots in order of size, all over the floor of the garage. He had probably been there all day.

The following morning, I went straight to the headmaster and told him of my decision. He was extremely sympathetic but left me in no doubt that I would have to work until the end of term, which also happened to be the end of the school year in July.

On the twenty-third of April 1985, my dear darling mother, who was so looking forward to me being at home with her, was taken into hospital, where she died. She was 88.

How's that for horrendous timing? I should have been there for her and I let her down. My wonderful, wonderful mother finished her life alone in a strange hospital surrounded by strangers. That is something that I will never, never forget.

12

Retirement, Reluctantly

In July 1985 it was my turn to leave the job that I had always
wanted since I was a child. I had very mixed feelings about it all.
The staff and the children were wonderful. Several parents who
had found out via the grapevine were also very supportive. They
came to the school or they sent 'good luck' and 'thank you'
messages via the children. They presumed I was taking normal
retirement and I was relieved about that. I don't think I could have
survived all the questions that I would have been subjected to had
they known I was retiring on compassionate grounds.

A week before the end of term I had the most wonderful party.
The first I knew about it was when I was asked whether I would
like a formal dinner at an hotel or an informal gathering in someone's home. I opted for the latter. In that way I would be able to
circulate and chat to everyone. It went without saying that Stan
was also invited and I knew he would prefer an informal setting.

Once I had expressed my views about that, the next question
really floored me. 'In that case, do you think we could possibly
have it at your house?'

I wondered if I had misheard and repeated, 'My house – did you
say my house?'

'It's just a thought but we hope you will agree. We have been
discussing it amongst ourselves and we thought it would be less of
a strain if Stan was in familiar surroundings. And you won't have
to do a thing. We will bring everything, food, drink – the lot. You
won't have to lift a finger, it will all be done by us. And we will
leave everything neat and tidy – we promise. Please say "Yes".'

They were so persuasive and I had to admit they were right. Our lounge would easily accommodate them and there were large patio doors into the garden. The kitchen would hold all the helpers without any problem. There was a large table in there and another in the dining room which was even bigger. And they were right about Stan. All he would have to do was relax and enjoy the fuss they would make of him.

And so it was arranged and it was marvellous! All the staff came, clerical as well as colleagues on the teaching staff. They brought along husbands and wives, girlfriends and boyfriends. And I was surprised and delighted to see some of my tutors from the training college who had also been invited.

The food and drink appeared as if by magic and disappeared just as quickly as everyone got into the party spirit. Stan's face was a picture. He was relaxed and smiling. It did me a world of good to see him looking so much at ease.

There were the inevitable speeches. The headmaster made a special point of saying how much he would miss my lovely northern accent. I secretly thought that had disappeared a long time ago!

There were flowers, cards, presents – and, at the end, nothing left for me to do. They were as good as their word and everything was put back into perfect order once again.

My only sadness was the comparison I couldn't help making between the way I was being treated and what it had been like for Stan just two years earlier. I couldn't bear to think about that and tried to blot it from my memory.

The last day of the school year was like all last days, hectic for the staff and a bit of a waste of time for the children. They were excited because they could bring games from home but, as usual, they soon got bored. Some of the things they had brought were highly unsuitable. Some were fragile and in danger of being broken, some were trivial beyond belief and only one or two had any educative value at all. But that final day was not the time for me to be critical. All I wanted was a bit of peace so that the room could be cleared and new stock put into place ready for the next school year. Stock for someone else, I thought – and a lump came into my throat. Some of the children pleaded with me to let them have a few of the old paints and some scraps of paper. Why not? I thought. The paint was only fit for throwing out.

Then it was lunch – an extended affair with a glass of wine. Soon it was time to return to the classroom for the last time.

The children were waiting with quiet anticipation for my return. Over the whole of the back wall display area were carefully painted letters which spelt out 'Thank you, Mrs Brown. We love you.' I was speechless and didn't know how I managed to keep back the tears. Then I turned to my desk. It was piled high with cards, parcels, flowers – oh, it was just like Christmas! And, just as at Christmas, I opened everything as expected and expressed my delight. I spent ages doing it and they watched my every move. It was lovely!

Assembly on the last day was always in the afternoon instead of first thing in the morning. I needed to brace myself for that. There was no way of playing the piano with eyes swimming with tears. I somehow survived the final 'thank-you' from the headmaster and the three cheers from the children. Then, for the last time, I played my own special version of the Lord's Prayer which the children loved to sing. They sang it beautifully.

And that was it. The end of the school year and the end of my career. Now all I had to do was devote my time to looking after Stan and get on with the rest of my life.

I took over my new role in life with very mixed feelings. There was an overwhelming relief in the fact that the decision had finally been made and I was now able to devote the whole of my time to tending to Stan's needs. But, as well as relief, there was also resentment. I wanted to shout out to the world at large and tell them how much giving up my job was affecting me, how much I was having to sacrifice, how much I was missing Mum and how fearful I was about the future.

But the strongest feeling of all was one of guilt. Why had I not been there when Mum needed me most? Why was I selfishly putting myself first when it was Stan who needed all the love and support that I could give? I was ashamed of myself and felt that I really did need to sort things out.

I was pleased to see how happy Stan was to have me around all day and he chatted away as though he hadn't a care in the world. He never mentioned the fact that he was no longer working and my hopes of him ever finding another job – any job, however trivial – had vanished long ago. I knew that the face he presented to the outside world was still one of normality. He looked much the same as he had always done. He was relaxed and cheerful – and he looked so young!

Friends and neighbours would greet us in the street and always the words were the same.

'Hello. My goodness, you look younger every day!'

It was Stan they were looking at. They couldn't say the same about me. I was disgusted with my appearance.

'How's retirement?'

Stan would always get in first with the answer.

'It's wonderful. Just being able to please yourself – no timetable to stick to. It's just great!'

His look at me conveyed the message – 'Don't you dare say anything else!'

And so, of course, I never did. If that was how Stan wanted it to be, then out of loyalty to him, I would stay silent.

Looking back at those early days of his illness, perhaps I was wrong to say nothing. Perhaps it would have been better all round had people realised that Stan was ill and that retirement for us both had not been out of choice. Apart from our family and close neighbours, no one knew that anything was amiss. Two years earlier, when Stan finished work, it was just accepted that he had been one of the lucky ones in the position to make that decision.

I was alone with a deep, dark secret that I couldn't speak about. Obviously, Gillian wondered and worried about us. But living in Berkshire and busy with two young boys, the younger one still only a few months old, she was unable to come and see us very often. Richard too, was preoccupied with his own affairs. He had just graduated from Newcastle University and was soon to embark on yet another course of studies for a further degree in agricultural engineering.

Meanwhile, as I have said, I was at home and Stan was delighted. Somehow we had to get back to some sort of normality.

I had no idea what to expect from his illness but, whilst Stan was still able, I wanted to make life as pleasant and varied as possible for us both. I was very apprehensive and wondered about my ability to cope. But this was it! Whatever fate had in store, I would have to be strong for both of us.

13

Taking Over the Reins

It wasn't long before the realisation dawned. Things were never going to be the same ever again and I had serious misgivings about being able to cope. But then, I had no alternative – somehow I would just have to take over the reins and try to keep things going just as smoothly as I could. It was a daunting prospect but hopefully I would be able to ease myself gently into my new rôle. I still couldn't believe that all this was happening. In any case, nothing drastic would happen straight away. Perhaps it never would, I told myself with false optimism.

But gradually, imperceptibly, the changes began. The first thing that worried me was his reluctance to deal with any post. It was just put to one side without even being opened. Letters were unanswered, bills remained unpaid. I just had to intervene.

'Are you going to open your letters?' I would ask.

His reply was usually just a grunt. Sometimes he would try to open the envelopes, usually making a complete mess in the attempt. More often than not he didn't even get to that stage and just completely forgot about them. I very soon knew that it was now up to me to deal with everything. It was as though my being at home had relieved him of all responsibilities. I was completely wrong in thinking that someone with his expertise would continue to deal with such mundane things as bills and accounts. I had thought that it would be a long time before he would be willing to let someone else deal with everything. But, here I was, much sooner than anticipated, being put to the test and expected to deal with everything.

Thank goodness for my banking experience was my one consoling thought. I already had authority to sign everything, so that was no problem. I took over the reins and he didn't even notice. I was horrified to realise that accountancy and management, which had formed a major part of his career, had become the first things to vanish from his mind. It was with a very heavy heart that I looked at him, just not able to believe this awful nightmare was happening. He looked so young and so very healthy – this just couldn't be happening.

Over and over again, I asked myself the same impossible questions. How would the disease progress? How much did he know about what was happening? How would he cope? How would I cope?

There were no answers. My mind was in a tumult and I suddenly felt that I had been presented with an insurmountable problem that wasn't going to go away. I needed to talk to somebody but knew of nobody who might understand.

That was the mental anguish. But, as the weeks and months went by, it was the day-to-day practicalities that had to take precedence. I gradually worked out a system to deal with each new problem as it arose. Very often it was a case of trial and error and I am certain that I made many errors along the way.

I tried to let him do things for himself, however long it took and however well or badly he did them. Many were the times he went out with what could only pass as an apology for a shave, and with just a cat-lick instead of a proper wash. He would put on whatever clothes he saw first – so I very quickly learnt to make sure only suitable ones were left where he could see them.

It was not long before I had to intervene and help with all of these things. I delayed for as long as possible as I knew that once I had helped he would never try on his own again.

Dressing was the first 'takeover'. He had no idea of the order of dressing – underpants on top of trousers somehow seemed quite acceptable to him. And, as for getting the right button into the correct buttonhole ... it was sheer luck when that happened. He began to have a phobia about anything going over his head – so jumpers were gradually replaced by cardigans, and to make life easier for me, buttons were replaced by zips.

As for shoes – oh dear – which foot should go into which shoe? Well at least he had a 50–50 chance of being right. Shoes were his bête noir – and he would accept my help – but never without stating a reason for needing help.

'I feel a bit stiff this morning' was his usual excuse.

Once I started to help with other items of clothing, that was it. I had the job for life.

It was at that stage that I had to work out a system for my own sanity.

First, his slippers. He would never go anywhere without something on his feet. So when I got him up in the mornings, that was my first job. Then it was a trip to the toilet and from there to the bathroom, next to it. I then had to persuade him to part with his pyjama top – quite difficult on some mornings – and wash the top half of him whilst he loudly protested with always the same words. 'What are you doing? Leave me alone. I never get dirty.'

Fortunately, he was continent and so it wasn't necessary to wash that part of his anatomy every day. He had to have a bath for me to make sure he was 'clean all over' and that was a mammoth undertaking requiring a lot of time and patience.

The next stage was to take him back into the bedroom and sit him down on a stand chair. This is where the crafty bit came in. As I was helping him to sit down, at the same time I would quickly remove his pyjama trousers – just far enough to make sure he wasn't sitting on them. The dressing could then be carried out in two simple stages. All the top half first – everything, including tie, cardigan or whatever was necessary, all sorted out the night before and all within arm's reach.

Then, with him still seated, it was underpants (just over his knees), trousers (the same), socks and finally shoes.

Then with just one final effort, I helped him to stand up and steady himself by holding on to my shoulders – and with one mighty heave, it was underpants up, trousers up, everything tucked in, all neat and tidy – and that was it!

Years later, when he was much worse, it somehow became easier. That was because he could never tell me whether he needed to sit or just stand at the toilet. So I played safe and always sat him down. It was comparatively easy then, to whip off both pyjama top and bottoms and then put all his things on whilst he was otherwise engaged. Admittedly, the wash he got was much less thorough – but my nervous exhaustion was kept at bay. He got plenty of baths anyway, so I wasn't worried.

So that was washing and dressing. And it was the same for everything else. I worked out a routine and then I stuck to it. Something must have registered with him, because if ever I deviated from this norm he would often begin to get upset and worried.

The only thing I never quite worked out was feeding him. I fed him at the kitchen table from a tray with non-slip mats, so the plates were always secure. I used a fork and spoon rather than a knife. I draped a huge napkin around him to keep him clean and made sure that anything that mattered was well out of his reach.

But the problem was me. Should I try to have my own meal at the same time? It could be very off-putting if he was in one of his 'baby' moods, playing with each mouthful before finally swallowing it. I decided it was probably easier for me to eat later, which meant reheating the meal. But more often than not, seeing Stan get into such a mess ruined my own appetite. Stan's appetite remained as good as ever whilst my own was rapidly disappearing.

I had to admit that in spite of me doing everything I could to keep everything 'normal' it was no longer working out that way. More and more, I was having to make decisions that would always have been left to Stan in the past. Before he became ill, he was always the dominant partner and that was the way I liked it, always happy to tag along.

But everything had changed. Take outings, for example. Everything in the past had always been organised by him. I would pack up a picnic lunch but that would be my sole contribution. Now, it was all up to me. I would wait for a fine day and then say, 'It's going to be lovely today. Shall we go out somewhere?'

'If you like.'

'Where would you like to go?'

'Anywhere.'

'How about you choosing somewhere today?'

'I don't know anywhere.'

'Of course you do. Come on, I like it when you choose.'

'Anywhere.'

The conversation having gone full circle, I was left with making my own decisions, which I hated. Then it would be the same about whether to pack up some food, which route to take – and so on. Stan was still driving. But I had to navigate. He relied on me completely.

The days out were rather strange, too. Gone were the days of mutual enjoyment, soaking up the history, the atmosphere, the ambience. Gone were the discussions, the exclamations and the oohs and ahs at each new discovery. He was there in body but the togetherness and the companionship had gone.

My poor Stan was finding it more and more difficult to keep going. Not a day went by without him saying 'I know I'm a mess and I'm so sorry. But I'm fighting it, you'll see, I'll not let it get the better of me.'

He really believed it and I encouraged him for all I was worth. If only I could have believed it too!

14

Ups and Downs

Three and a half years had passed since that fateful day in 1983 when Stan had become 'surplus to requirements'. He was valiantly trying to get the most out of life and we tried to get out and about as much as possible. I could detect signs that things were very gradually deteriorating but I firmly believed that I was the only one who would notice.

The caravan had had to go. There was no way that caravan holidays would feature in our lives again. We did manage a brief holiday in Somerset with Peggy and Syd. We each of us took our own caravan. But Stan needed so much help. Syd was having to sort him out continually, I was on tenterhooks all the time and it really wasn't worth all the hassle. I was dreadfully upset about it as caravanning had been our way of life for so many years. Of course, in Stan's eyes, I was everything that was horrible! I was a deceitful, wicked and cruel woman – just about the worst person on earth.

Things were not running quite so smoothly at home either. Stan continued to answer the phone if I was not around. The trouble was that he never remembered to pass on any messages. I got into hot water time and time again by my apparent indifference about what had been said to him. A notepad and pencil by the phone were completely ignored. In any case I doubted his ability to write down any messages – ironically it was his writing skills that were the first to disappear. And leaving the phone off the hook only irritated the callers, who simply didn't understand. It was many years later when the problem solved itself – he didn't know where to

J Brown

14 Sutcliffe

got walke in Worcester

R & Jill went wit

uth to jet a Parl

of water

Jack and brok his
Cro

The ability to write was one of Stan's first skills to go.

find the phone. Now, of course, I have an answerphone – but they weren't around when I needed one.

I remember one dreadful day when he failed to turn up to collect me from a Christmas party. It was in the neighbouring village of Kempsey where I was treasurer of the WI. It was an afternoon affair and he had taken me along and knew he had to collect me at around 4.30 p.m. I had written him a big notice, which he was annoyed about because he said he didn't need it. Anyway, because I had gone by car, I didn't bother to put a coat on, or gloves, or scarf.

At 4.30 everyone started to leave. 'Are you OK? Have you a lift?'

I assured everyone that Stan would be along any minute and they all disappeared. But there was no sign of Stan. I tried to phone him. This time, I really did want him to answer – but there was no reply. Was that because he was on his way? I had no means of finding out. I decided I had better set off to walk the three miles home. If I faced the oncoming traffic, hopefully he would see me. I was dazzled by all the headlights and couldn't see a thing. I had no coat and it was freezing. I was wearing the most unsuitable high-heeled shoes and I was trying to carry, in frozen, gloveless hands, a whole pile of things – cash (all silver and copper and weighing a ton), plates and dishes and a stupid Christmas table decoration which I had been asked to make for one of the tables. Then, it began to snow. That was it! The stupid thing finished up behind someone's hedge. I often wonder if they ever found it! Suddenly the hard pavement disappeared and my heels were sinking into the soft grass verge with every step. Never had three miles felt to be such a long way.

When I finally arrived home, there was Stan sitting in the dark in the lounge.

'Where have you been?' was his greeting. And before I could answer, he added 'It's dark and I'm hungry.'

At the beginning of 1987, I had the most wonderful surprise. Coming back from shopping, I heard the phone ringing as I opened the door. I managed to get to it before it stopped ringing and heard a voice say 'Hello, is that Mrs Audrey Brown?'

'Yes?' I answered questioningly.

'This is Mensa, Wolverhampton. I am ringing to let you know that you have won the "Mind Games" competition. Congratulations!'

I was speechless. It seemed ages since I had sent off my entry and I had forgotten all about it.

The voice continued, 'Your prize is a break for two people in Washington, DC.'

I managed to say something. I hope it was 'thank you' but my mind was racing. I was so excited. I had never ever won anything in my life before, with the exception of a set of towels in a raffle at a fashion show, which I received from no less a person than Michael Aspel. That, to date, had been my one moment of glory.

The voice explained that I had solved all 60 problems correctly and, along with the other correct entries, the limerick tie-breakers had been discussed by the Mensa Board. I remember Richard reading it before I sent off the entry and his derision. 'That will never win anything,' was all he said. I was inclined to agree with him. But perhaps it was just because it was so stupid that it was chosen.

> There was a young man from New York
> Who pierced three balloons with a fork.
> He found they were chewy
> When mixed with chop suey
> And wished he had settled for pork.

I was then informed that they would be sending me all the details and would I make sure our passports were in order and arrange to get visas.

I put the phone down in a daze.

'What's wrong?' Stan was by my side. Phone calls no longer meant anything to him and he took no notice. But this time something had registered. Perhaps it was my face!

'Nothing. There's nothing wrong. I've won a prize. We've won a trip to America!'

His face was a picture. He was trying to take it all in. It hadn't really registered with me yet, so I knew how mixed up he was bound to be.

'Let's go and tell Peggy and Syd. Come on, let's go now!' I had to go and talk to someone rational.

Our neighbours were thrilled for us and thought it was fantastic. We chatted non-stop. They had friends over in America and could tell us a lot about what to expect. But, gradually, as the initial excitement subsided, common sense began to take over. Peggy, always the practical one, wondered just how I was going to manage.

'You'll have all the responsibility. Will you cope?'

I was far from sure. We had neither of us ever flown before. We had had holidays on the Continent – France, Austria, Germany, Switzerland – but always with the caravan, which meant a sea crossing. So this would be a first for us both. We would be there for a full week and I would have to take charge of everything. Was it going to mean anything to Stan? Would it be too much for him? Would we be able to get out and about?

During the next few weeks, I thought of little else. It was Stan himself who finally helped me to make up my mind. He talked about it. He mentioned it on several occasions. So it had registered and, bless him, he deserved to go.

The decision was made and the preparations began.

On the nineteenth of March 1987, on a bitterly cold day, we drove to our daughter's in Bracknell and stayed there overnight. And the following morning, Jeremy took us to Heathrow Airport to catch BA flight 217 from Terminal Four, leaving at 11.45 a.m. And so began the most memorable week of our lives.

It was the beginning of a whole set of new experiences for me and I truly believe it meant a lot to Stan too. We watched the ribbon of the River Thames disappear beneath fluffy white clouds and then everything was blue – brilliant and permanent. We sipped Tia Maria, ate honey-roast chicken and saw *Crocodile Dundee*.

At last came the information from the pilot that I had been waiting for. Below us was the St Lawrence Seaway. We could see huge ice floes. And then it was the Eastern seaboard and eventually a long descent to Dulles Airport. Once through the customs, we were taken by a sort of 'minibus' – The Washington Flyer – to downtown Washington. I thought of how cold it was in England. But, here, spring had arrived and everyone was smiling. There were daffodils everywhere, the magnolias were magnificent and the famous cherry trees were just beginning to blossom. Temperatures stayed in the high sixties, just perfect for sightseeing and picnics on the Mall. We 'did' Washington in true tourist style – we even saw President Reagan getting into his helicopter on the White House lawn. We were thrilled with our visits to the White House, the Smithsonian Museums, the Kennedy Center, Arlington, Georgetown and the art museums. Washington was a marvellous place for strolling, especially in the beautiful weather that lasted throughout our visit. The Air and Space Museum was fantastic and we were thrilled to see for ourselves Lindbergh's *Spirit of St Louis* and the Wright Brothers' *Flyer*. We walked inside Skylab and marvelled at the smallness of John Glenn's space capsule. We enjoyed a tour of Washington on 'The Old Trolley-bus' and saw the former and present houses of such people as Jacqueline Kennedy, 'Wonder Woman', George Bush, Henry Kissinger, Alexander Graham Bell. We saw Ford's Theatre, where Lincoln met his end, and the infamous Watergate Hotel.

Stan was amazing. He took it all in his stride and for quite a long time after our return would talk about his trip to America. I am so glad I plucked up the courage to take him.

15

More Holiday Times

The years dragged on and on with every day full of all sorts of problems. There were very few red-letter days when something of note happened to relieve the monotony. Christmas 1992 was no different to any other time of the year. We were not going anywhere and if the family did manage to come it would not be until well into the New Year. It was welcome therefore, when Peggy and Syd decided to go down to relatives in Brighton towards the end of January 1993 – just for a few days, but if we wanted, they would take us to Gillian's and collect us again on the way back. So, on the twenty-first of January, we found ourselves in Bracknell. It was hard work keeping tabs on Stan but it was worth it. It was great to be with them for a few days and greater still to have some relief from caring as Gillian helped as much as possible.

It was just for a few wonderful days and then, on the following Sunday – the twenty-fourth – Peggy and Syd brought us back to Worcester again. It was grand to have the help and support of such good friends and neighbours. Imagine the absolute horror and shock, therefore, when just four days later – on the Thursday – without warning, Peggy suddenly collapsed and died. Poor Syd was so devastated, the whole neighbourhood was in deep shock and we had just lost the very best friend that anyone could ever have. I can remember ringing Gillian with the news and her disbelief – 'She can't have died, she was sitting on our settee having a cup of coffee only a couple of days ago. Mum, it just can't be true!'

But it was, and things could never ever be the same again. Syd was inconsolable; Stan knew that something was wrong but couldn't grasp just what we all looked so sad about. For a time, my worries had to take a back seat as everyone tried to do something to help Syd. What a sad beginning to the year!

The twentieth of May 1993. Stan's sixty-seventh birthday. Ten years had gone by since that fateful day when our lives changed forever. I looked back with nostalgia at all the things we used to do, at all the plans we made and at all the dreams we had about our future. We should have reached that time in our lives when all our dreams and all our hopes should be coming true.

But the reality was now so very different. None of our dreams have materialised. None were ever possible as the dreadful disease moved relentlessly on. It moved at its own rate and took its own time – in Stan's case it was so very slowly, almost imperceptibly – but the deterioration was there. The disease was destroying little bits of him every day.

He depended on me for so much. I had gradually taken over all the things that used to be his domain and he didn't even notice. For many years, as well as Alzheimer's Disease, he has had so much trouble with his eyesight. The problems started way back in 1985 when we were on holiday in Saundersfoot and have got steadily worse ever since. There has been so much that he has had to cope with. And with each little downward step, I have had to be there to make his pathway as smooth as possible.

It was on his sixty-seventh birthday that I decided to keep a diary. I am still writing notes in it today – any special happenings, any moments of nostalgia, all the good things and all traumatic moments that have caused so much distress.

On his sixty-seventh birthday, we were actually in Saundersfoot again. This time we were on holiday with Richard and Joy. We were staying in a luxury caravan on our very special site where we had been many times before. What I didn't know then, was it would be Stan's last visit here.

'Happy birthday, Dad!' Richard handed him a parcel and a card.

Stan didn't know it was his birthday, even though it was less than a minute since I had also given him his present and a card. He looked mildly surprised and then, as he very often did, put on a

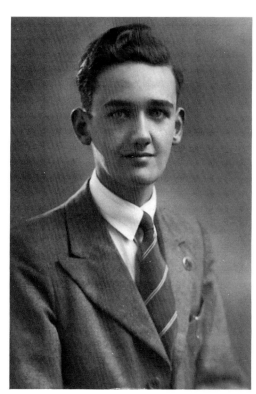

Stan – not quite 18 years old.

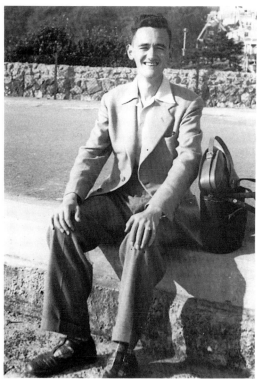

Stan – at Thorpe Bay, Essex – 1948.
He was 22 – we were engaged.

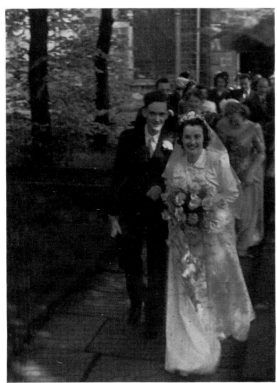

Our wedding. 3 June 1950.
Informal photograph.

Our wedding. The 'official' one.

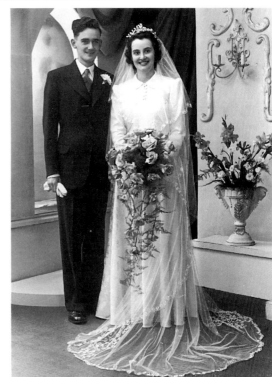

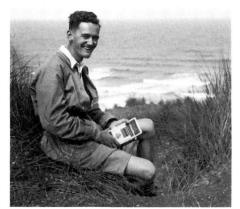

June 1953. Stan – Perranporth, Cornwall.
Just one of our many walking holidays.

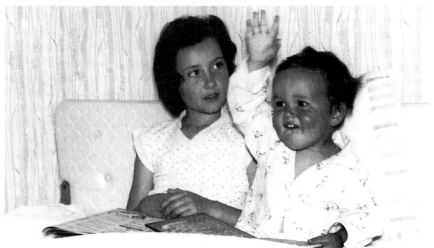

Late '64 or early '65 – our two children – early morning – both in one bed!!

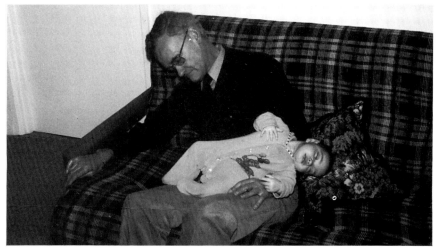

Late '82 – before I really knew he was ill, although all the signs were there. Stan is 'baby-sitting'! Simon, our grandson, is only a few weeks old.

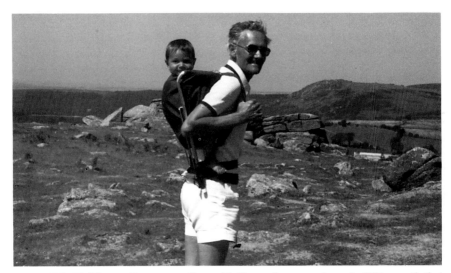

August '83. Walking on Dartmoor – Stan with Simon. It was at the end of this month that Stan's working days came to a close – he was 57.

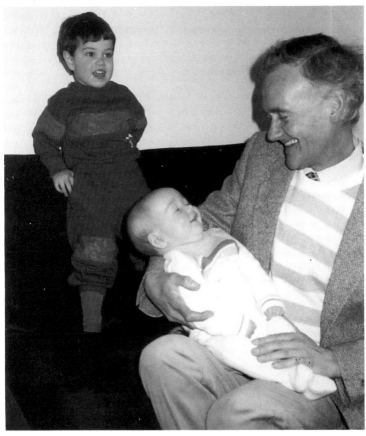

Both grandchildren with their grandad. Simon (born 7/10/82) and Richard (born 15/12/84). The picture was taken early 1985.

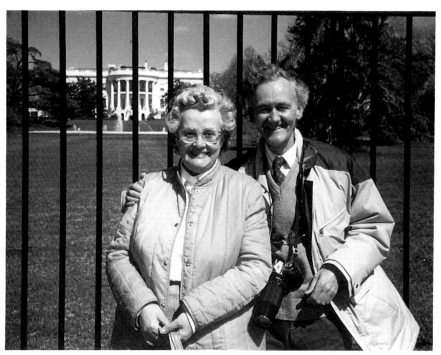

March 1987. The White House, Washington DC. How did I find the courage to go?

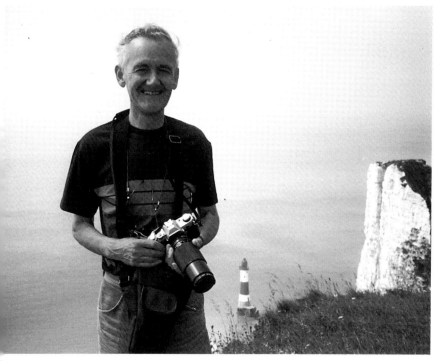

Still 1987 – Beachy Head – late summer – he had started to wander – causing many extra problems.

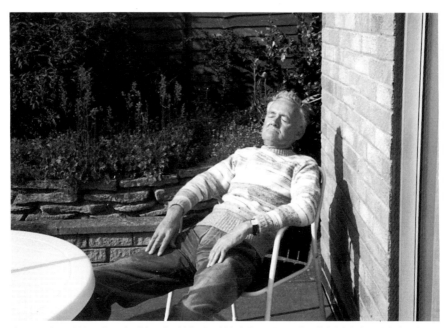

Our garden 1989 – Stan had just had his 63rd birthday. He really did think he still did all the gardening.

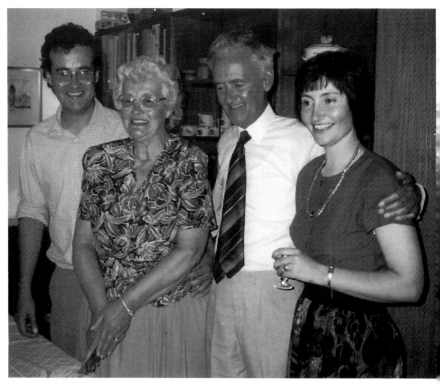

A photo taken at our Ruby wedding. He doesn't appear to ail a thing, does he? No wonder people didn't believe I had any problems!

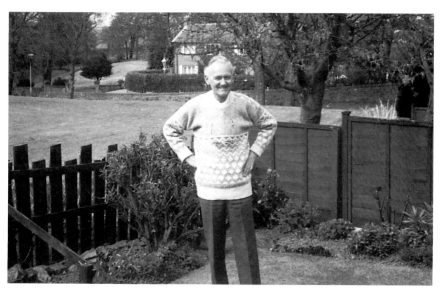

April '91. Stan is still not quite 65. The photo is at his sister's house (Doreen & Frank) in Lancashire. Their view of the Pennines is superb! This was Stan's last visit – I couldn't cope any longer with the journey.

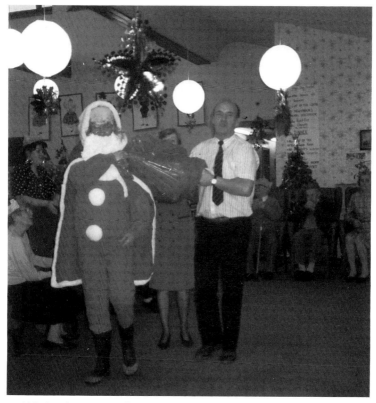

Christmas '91. Stan is now attending the Elgar Day Centre – he is very disabled and confused. (He makes a very slim Father Christmas!)

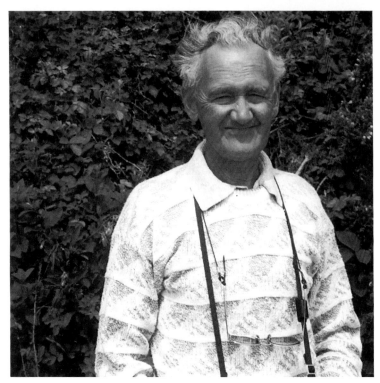

May '92 (almost 66 years old). On holiday with Peggy and Syd at Saundersfoot. The camera and spectacles went everywhere with him – but neither were of any use to him.

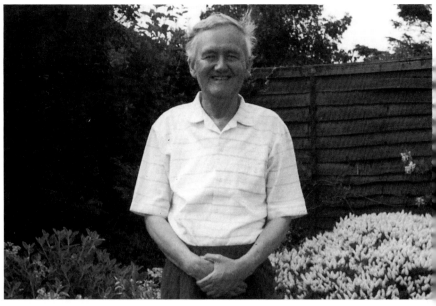

The last photograph I have of Stan before he went into a nursing home – taken in our garden, summer '94. He is 68. The following March he became so ill that a nursing home was my only option. He went to Welland House on 13/3/95.

great act in order to convince everybody that he knew all the time about his birthday.

'Thank you. You shouldn't have bothered.' Both card and parcel remained unopened.

'Shall I help you, Dad?' Richard reached over and opened his card. 'There you are,' he said, handing it over.

'What's this then?'

'It's a birthday card from us both.'

'Oh, that's nice. Is it my birthday?'

With great patience, Richard once more quietly told him that it was and that he was 67.

'Sixty-seven. Is that right? Well, I don't know.'

He took the card from Richard but couldn't read it. Richard read it out to him and then, one by one, we showed him the others – from Gillian, the grandchildren, friends, neighbours, other relatives and the one from me.

We displayed the cards in the caravan and made a ceremony of opening his presents. We had a special birthday breakfast and we made a great fuss of him.

We were rewarded with some lovely smiles, but Stan still didn't know it was his birthday.

After breakfast, Richard drove us to Solva, where he and Joy went for a long cliff walk and Stan and I sat enjoying the beautiful scenery and the peace. We had lunch in Solva and then went to St David's and finally to St Justinian, which was new territory for us and very enjoyable. I would have enjoyed a long walk with Richard and Joy but knew it would not be possible for Stan.

Two days later, it was time to return to Worcester after a lovely break. I think Stan had enjoyed it although it was always hard to judge from his expressions. The activity before we left the site was obviously worrying him. He knew something was happening but the reason for all the packing up, sorting out the car and going to the site office to settle the account was completely beyond his comprehension.

Then he was worried all the way home. 'Where are we going? What's happening? Nobody ever tells me anything.'

Back home again, he was completely disorientated as I had expected him to be. But by the time I had finished the essentials that arriving home always entailed and Richard and Joy had left, he was once again sitting quietly in his favourite chair and all memories of the holiday, the caravan, the journey home, the time spent with Richard and Joy, everything, had vanished forever.

The very next day was the start of another very worrying time for him. Gillian and the family had arranged to come over. It was the start of their annual holiday and I had agreed to look after Peter, their little dog, whilst they were abroad. I wasn't worried about Peter. He was a lovely dog and very fond of his 'grandma'. But, I was worried about Stan's reactions. Peter was quite an elderly little poodle and his needs were few – a nice full tummy, walks, access to the garden and plenty of love and affection. From being a puppy, there had been a bond between Stan and Peter. But now, things were different. Stan was worried and irritated whilst Peter, with what I was convinced was an animal sixth sense, carefully avoided contact with him and growled whenever Stan was anywhere near him.

I was left with the full time care of both of them. With Stan's very poor vision and Peter's tendency to get under the feet, I had to be constantly vigilant to prevent any accidents. Access to the garden for Peter also meant an escape route for Stan. I didn't think he would realise that but, nevertheless, I had to keep tabs on them both.

One day I had a dental appointment. The surgery is only a matter of two or three minutes' walk away from our bungalow, but I still felt uneasy about leaving the two of them alone together.

'You'll stay in, won't you? I shan't be long.' Whatever made me say that, I'll never know. Stan was having so much difficulty in getting about that he never went anywhere without my help.

After my appointment, I rushed home. Please, please let everything be all right was my only thought.

As I went in, Peter rushed to meet me and Stan was sitting in his usual chair.

Thank goodness, I thought. And I relaxed.

The following day, Jim called to me over the fence. 'Is everything all right?' I assured him that it was. Jim then continued 'I was just a bit worried about yesterday. Didn't Stan tell you?'

'Tell me – tell me what?'

86

'Oh dear, perhaps I shouldn't have said anything – but...' He hesitated and then continued. 'But I was so worried when I saw Stan and the dog walking down Bath Road. I was in the car and I stopped and asked him if he wanted a lift. I was worried because he looked strange.'

My heart was pounding. 'Never – how on earth had he got into Bath Road? Was Peter on his lead?'

'Oh yes,' Jim confirmed. 'But I'm glad I stopped because he told me he was lost and he was so relieved when he saw me.'

'Oh, Jim,' I said, 'thank goodness you did stop. I had no idea... I didn't know he'd been out.'

'Didn't he say anything?' said Jim. 'I never thought to come round. I watched him go into your house – the back door was wide open so I knew you were in.'

My mind was in a whirl. Thank goodness Jim had spotted him. How on earth had Stan managed to find Peter's lead and put it on him? How had he managed to walk unaided to the very busy main road? What a good thing Jim had stopped and brought him home. The back door was closed when I came home. Stan must have done that – and taken Peter's lead off again and put it back where he had found it.

I just couldn't believe it. I thought it was all beyond Stan's capabilities and but for Jim, it was something I would never have known about ... unless (I went cold) ... unless the outcome had been very different and they had come to grief.

The days of looking after Peter continued and were now really worrying me.

'Why is Peter here?' If Stan asked that question once he must have repeated it umpteen times over.

One evening, I was watering the bedding plants and was suddenly shocked to see Peter dash straight past me and into the road. He'd got out because Stan had opened the drive gates. His new-found freedom could have spelt disaster but, fortunately for me, he was diverted by all the new smells that needed investigating and I quickly caught up with him and returned him to safety. As I closed the gates, I turned to Stan and asked him why he had opened them and got the reply, 'I thought you might want to take the watering can into the street.'

I resisted the temptation to ask him why he thought I would want to do that. Instead, I asked him if he would like to help by filling the can again for me.

'I will if I can find the tap.' He took the lid off the dustbin and looked surprised when there wasn't a tap there.

Without thinking, I said, 'No. You won't find any water there. Let me show you.'

That was enough for him. The can was thrown at me with full force. 'Do it yourself!' he shouted, and then went indoors, slamming the door behind him.

I finished the watering and then went indoors to join him.

'Would you like a drink?' I asked.

'Oh yes please. You are kind.' He gave me a lovely smile. How could I possibly be cross with him?

16

A Month of Muddles and Upsets

The following Sunday started off very badly. For the first time ever, I hadn't heard Stan get up during the night and, even more surprisingly – as far as I know – neither had Peter. He had gone into the bathroom instead of the toilet and when I got up I found the floor, bath mat and towels soaking wet. I prayed that this wasn't going to be yet another downward step for him.

During the morning, Syd called and took us over to our friends Fay and Mike for coffee. Stan was very quiet, in fact I don't think he spoke at all. I felt hurt that he was being ignored whilst Peter was getting a great deal of fuss. I suppose that I am becoming hypersensitive about the way other people are reacting to him.

Monday was no better. Stan tried to dismantle one of the taps in the washbasin. I was still trying to encourage him to do as much as he could for himself but it was really hard going. The trouble was that once I took over and started to help him he then thought I would keep on doing it for evermore. The day continued as it had started. He made an awful mess with his breakfast, which he declared was rubbish. He grumbled about his socks, his shoes, his teeth, his electric shaver – everything!

In the afternoon, Olive and Jim took us to a garden centre – they needed more bedding plants and so did I. But this time, even with my help, Stan was unable to negotiate the path from the car to the garden area and I had to go back with him and wait with him in the car. How on earth had he managed his walk with Peter? I still can't believe it.

In the evening, we settled down to watch television. Again, this was becoming another minefield for me as I never knew how he would react. There was a lovely nature programme, but all at once Stan became so disturbed and upset by it that I had to switch the set off.

The following Tuesday was an Elgar Centre day and, as usual, I was up by seven o'clock in order to have Stan ready. This was something else that was fraught with problems. On a bad day, I needed the whole time to make sure Stan was ready before the transport arrived. But if it was one of his good days, I only needed half that time and then he had an hour at least in which to get himself into a mess and completely 'unready' again.

However, on this particular Tuesday it was even worse than usual. The transport never arrived! I was just about to explode when I suddenly remembered the date. It was the first of June – the day after Whit Monday. There wouldn't be any day care.

I was usually sent a reminder – but this time there hadn't been anything. Oh what a clot I was. If I allowed it, it could have been enough to put me in a bad mood for the rest of the day.

When the post arrived, there was the June Newsletter from the Alzheimer's Disease Society, which also contained disturbing reading. Perhaps this is the place to write about it – get things off my chest, once and for all, and then try to get on with living.

The Newsletter contained a long letter from the Editor commenting on some of the offensive journalism which seemed to be attacking carers. He also condemned the *Panorama* programme entitled 'Dumping Granny', which labelled carers as some sort of beasts who beat, torment, rob and 'put away' relatives rather than allow them to become a nuisance. Carers seem to be becoming the scapegoats of the new community care system. The reality is rather different. The government does not seem to be finding the money, the health services seem to be opting out and social workers are not able to meet all the needs. It appears, therefore, that it is becoming a case of 'Don't blame any of the official bodies. Just blame the carers.'

I felt so depressed when I read all this. All I have ever wanted to do was to help Stan in every way possible. That was why I finished work. I never once counted the cost of doing so. I wanted to be there for him when he needed me. I wanted him to have as good a quality of life as possible. Those were, and still are my feelings and I am sure they are the feelings of so many carers throughout the country.

But the article made me think. Through no fault of our own, we were paying a colossal price. We had just, willingly and proudly, paid for the best education possible for our children when the blow fell and almost overnight our incomes almost disappeared. Our income came from pensions from work, which were derisory, and unemployment benefit. When that benefit finished it was replaced by a disability allowance. And that was it.

But it wasn't the money that affected us most. It was so many other things. Stan was still so young but I very soon found out that what he was suffering from was treated as something that happened in old age. There was no way that I could even begin to get over the message that Stan's needs were very different to someone many years his senior. For people of his age, there was absolutely no provision at all. There are statistics available showing that only one person in a thousand below the age of 65 will have Alzheimer's Disease. Stan was one of those unfortunate people – and the powers that existed in 1983 when Stan was only 56 didn't recognise that younger people did not fit easily into the slot provided for much older people.

Even now, the younger people are still badly off compared to the rest. For us, therefore, we counted the cost in terms of loss of freedom, loss of years of retirement to which we had both been looking forward and which have now just become a 'nothingness'. There was the loss of friends who suddenly became embarrassed and stayed away, loss of hope, loss of any sense of purpose in life, and loss of a real sense of humour. For me it also meant loss of sleep, which was replaced by a perpetual tiredness, depression and worry. If only people could understand, just have an inkling of what had happened to us.

In the evening, as I was getting him ready for bed, he said, 'Where are we? What's happening? Are you staying with me?'

I replied, 'We're at home and of course I'm staying with you.'

'Oh, thank goodness! Don't ever leave me, will you?' He gripped my arm tightly and repeated the same words.

Two days later it was our forty-third wedding anniversary but I

91

was the only one who remembered. Poor Stan would be so upset if he realised. Our anniversaries had always been something special until his illness. It was just another ordinary, tiring and rather boring day. As usual, I tried to do too much and I was exhausted.

Sunday, 6 June – Stan was out of bed for the umpteenth time. He couldn't need the toilet, he'd only just been. I looked at the clock – it was three o'clock.

'Come back to bed. It's too early to get up.' Reluctantly he agreed.

At four o'clock he was up again. 'What are you doing?' I asked.

'Just making a cup of tea,' was his reply. There was nothing else for it. I got him back into bed and then went into the kitchen to boil the kettle. And there we were, at quarter past four in the morning, sat up in bed having our first drink of the day. Peter was grumpy. He didn't like being disturbed at this ridiculous hour.

'Are we having to pay for Peter in this hotel?' asked Stan. And that question answered, he then went on, 'Do I owe you ten shillings?' Whenever he mentioned money, it was always the old currency.

He spotted his sandals by the dressing table. 'Look at my shoes. They're full of holes,' and then, as I took his empty cup from him, 'Have we had our dinner yet?'

I tried to persuade him to lie down again. 'I shan't have another cup of tea here.'

I should have just agreed with him. Instead I asked him why not.

'Well, I'm going home today.'

'So why don't you try and have a sleep before you have to get ready?'

'Are you going home, too?'

'I shall stay with you.'

'Oh, that's all right, then.'

His eyes finally closed and he was asleep.

June turned out to be quite a month of downward steps. The toilet problem got worse. He was still able to indicate when he needed it but could no longer find the right place. For a long time there had been a notice and a picture of a toilet on the door. But now, he neither saw it nor recognised it if he happened to spot it. I therefore had to be particularly vigilant and watch for all the signs. I then had to take him to the right place, make sure he was OK and then leave him his bit of privacy. I then had to sort him out afterwards. There was no way he could clean himself up (if that was necessary) and if he had only spent a penny, I needed to check the toilet, as (not to put too fine a point on it) his aim was erratic to say the least. Thank goodness, I had dispensed with a carpet in the toilet many years earlier and the tiles were easy to keep clean.

June was also the month when he literally gave up when it came to eating. He couldn't (or wouldn't) use the cutlery and it was therefore up to me to do everything for him. His appetite was good but he no longer made any attempt to feed himself.

It was the same with his appearance. Always very meticulous about how he looked, he suddenly lost all interest. I took over everything, including shaving, which I hated because he always made such a fuss.

'It's just like looking after a baby,' said those who knew nothing.

I would just nod – but I was incensed by their remark and would have loved to reply 'It's nothing at all like looking after a baby. It's exactly the opposite. The delight of watching a tiny, helpless baby learn new skills and slowly develop into an adorable toddler can never be compared to the heartache of watching my wonderful husband become more and more dependent on me and literally disintegrating day by day.'

June was a month of muddles and upsets.

'How much longer will they let me stay with you? How long are you staying here?' He would ask these questions, often with tears in his eyes, and I never knew what to say. I wanted to ask him if he knew anything about what was happening to him – but of course I couldn't. There were days when I felt certain that he had some inkling of what was going on – they were dreadful days and I felt so inadequate and unable to console him. On other days, he seemed completely oblivious of anything. I felt that those days were better for him but my own sadness was unbearable.

June was the month when he began to see things that weren't there. He would crawl around the floor, picking up 'things' that only he could see. He would think he was at a football match or on a train. He would accuse me of stealing his money and hiding his belongings.

One day, he spent ages moving his head round and round and round. When I asked him what he was doing, his answer was 'I'm just stirring that thing up.'

He didn't know who he was. He didn't know where he was. But, worst of all, he didn't always know who I was.

June was the month I decided that never again could I ever leave him on his own, not even for a minute.

It was also the month when the staff at the Elgar Centre realised I needed more help and were trying to arrange a few days' respite care. Eventually, Keith, his personal nurse, rang me to say that West Wing would look after him for a few days. August was the first date available – just from Thursday the fifth until Monday the ninth. I thanked him, put the phone down and collapsed in tears.

It was what I needed. It was meant to help me – but it was just another downward step. What could I be thinking of in allowing him to go? I looked at him, settled and comfortable and thought, of course I can manage – he's fine.

That evening, he settled down quickly and had a good night. I never slept a wink!

17

Respite

The following day started at six o'clock. That wasn't bad but, as if to prove a point, the trouble then started. Everything I did was wrong. I was told to leave him alone. He shouted and swore at me, and his cries were accompanied by punches to my chest and kicks to my legs. His breakfast was pronounced as rubbish, as was his lunch. He resisted all attempts by me to make him more comfortable. Classic FM, which he usually loved, was upsetting him, so it had to go off. The television was an even bigger menace. So that, too, went off.

I found myself with tears in my eyes for the smallest of reasons. I was so depressed and thought that perhaps I really was cracking up.

It was a beautiful day and we seemed to be the only ones around. Olive and Jim had gone off to the cricket at the county ground. Syd was obviously out and there was no sign of any of our other neighbours. I felt isolated and alone.

Ah well, at least the tennis from Wimbledon was good and Stan slept all through it.

The time for Stan to go into West Wing was getting closer and I still had very mixed feelings about it. Gillian, bless her, knew how I was feeling and they had decided to take me away for a few days whilst he was in respite care. I wasn't sure if that was what I really wanted. In fact, I was so mixed up about everything – it was quite unlike me to be so confused. I still hadn't mentioned West Wing to Stan – I wasn't sure whether I should or not.

The next day, Monday, the fifth of July, was the beginning of

Alzheimer's Awareness Week. Stan listened, or appeared to listen, to a short news item about it and I plucked up courage and mentioned West Wing. 'It will only be for a few days,' I said.

'Good idea,' was all he said. But my conscience was eased and I felt as though a load had been lifted from my mind.

It was another of his muddled days. He didn't know where to get off the train. And 'Why are all those people dashing about?'

I tried to tell him to stop worrying and he was suddenly in tears.

'I'll be all right. Just as long as I can see you.'

I started to worry about respite care, all over again!

At the beginning of August, Stan went into West Wing. Common sense told me that I was doing the right thing. But my heart was so heavy as I watched the ambulance turn the corner of the street and disappear from view. Gillian and the family arrived and, after an emotional meeting, we left for a few days in Devon. The hotel, on Dartmoor, was wonderful and so was the weather. It took me some considerable time to unwind and Stan was never far from my thoughts. This was the first time I had ever gone away without him, and now, here I was doing all the things he used to love – long walks on the moors and lovely relaxing times on the beaches. I was so sad, but my batteries were being recharged and I would hopefully be ready to take over the reins again on my return.

Stan was confused and disorientated when we went to collect him on the following Monday morning. He registered a mixture of emotions including excitement and tears. I knew this was a first of what would probably be many more days for him in West Wing. I also knew that I would never be happy to see him go – but it was the only chance to unwind that I was being offered and for both our sakes I knew that that was what I must be prepared to do.

The following day, when Stan awoke, his first words were 'Have I been in prison?'

I teased him, and asked him what he had done wrong.

'It must have been a dream.'

I agreed and he seemed satisfied.

Later on, he said, 'Where's my driving licence?'

'You don't drive any more, so you don't need one.'

'What if I start driving again?'

'You won't be able to because of your eyes.' I couldn't say anything about his mind.

'Where's my car?'

'We sold it a long time ago.'

'Why don't we sell those boxes?'

'Which boxes?'

He pointed to our wardrobes and I tried to explain to him what they were but he looked more confused.

'Will we take them when we go?'

'Go? Where do you think we have to go?'

'Home.'

'We are at home.'

Stan looked round in complete bewilderment – and then, looking straight at me, said, 'Excuse me. Who are you?'

I was completely shocked and tried, in vain, to help him to remember my name. It was no use and I was devastated. In the end, I had to tell him.

'That's funny. I used to know somebody called Audrey.' Then he continued, 'Where were you born?'

'Nelson,' I replied.

'Well, I don't know! That's where I was born! Do you know my sisters?'

'Yes. They are called Edith and Doreen.'

'Oh dear. I hope you aren't frightened of them. Are we on a train?'

'No.'

'Oh. I'm glad.' With that, he settled down in bed and closed his eyes. I left him resting peacefully whilst I got up and prepared myself for the normal morning marathon which would soon have to begin.

It all started again when I went to get him up.

'I shall be glad to leave this place. It's full of yobs.'

'I think you've been dreaming again.'

'They've gone quiet now – but not for long. They'll be back.'

I started to get him up and for once, he didn't resist.

'Are we going home?' I tried to tell him that he was at home.

'Oh yes. This is where I live, isn't it? When are you going?'

'I live here with you. Do you know who I am?'

He looked straight at me and said, 'You're Audrey. Don't leave me, will you?' and his eyes filled with tears.

'Of course I won't. This is where I live as well.'

'Oh. I didn't know.'

Later, when the transport arrived to take him to the day centre, he turned to me with great concern and told me that he had to go and that I would be here on my own.

'Will you be all right? Will you be able to manage?'

He arrived home in a terrible state. Someone had taken his anorak (he was actually wearing it), he'd lost all his money, he hadn't had anything to eat, they'd all gone out and left him on his own and now they had just dumped him here.

'Why,' he wanted to know, 'won't they let me go home?'

18

The Final Straw

The summer continued. Life was following some sort of crazy routine that I no longer felt to have any control over. In the quiet moments, I would make plans that at the time seemed sensible. But I was finding that frequently those same plans had to be abandoned as I gave way to Stan's moods and behaviour far removed from rational thought.

On the good days, if I rang Gillian, she would know immediately from my voice that things were fine – it registered in my voice and she didn't need to ask. Sometimes, I was able to pass the phone over to Stan and he would speak to her. Never for long, never with anything sensible to say, but she would listen and be reassured. But I was very much aware that the good days were getting rather scarce.

It was August and I watched with envy as our neighbours busied themselves with 'normal' activities – picnics, exciting excursions with the children still on holiday from school, a quiet time in the garden or an outing in the car. By contrast, the highlight of our day would probably be planning a walk to our local Tesco's. I don't think 'excitement' was quite the right word, but it had to be just as carefully planned and it was taking more and more courage on my part to carry out all the strategic manoeuvres. Today had been one of my brave days. I managed to get Stan there and back without incident and I even managed to buy all the things on my list.

But the following day was different. It was a bad day that started at half-past five. Stan was worried about missing his train.

He wouldn't be able to give me any money for looking after him. His mother didn't look after him properly and he hadn't got any clothes to wear. Worst of all, he had lost all the things he needed to eat with – whatever did he mean? Surely he didn't mean his teeth!

Thank goodness it was a Saturday. I would never have got him ready for day care. It was almost lunchtime before I got him to settle down. I thought he was dozing until he suddenly opened his eyes and said, 'Why don't you give me a couple of pills to finish me off?' There were tears in his eyes as he said it, which made me cry, too. Whatever must have been going on to make him say something like that? What a horrible, horrible thought.

I sat with him for ages, talking quietly to him, stroking him, caressing him, trying to make him feel happy again. At last he calmed down. He again looked straight at me and said with such feeling, 'Why won't you let me go home? I've lost Audrey.'

He was really upsetting me and I just didn't know what to say. Perhaps music might help. It usually worked for a time. I began to play the piano and soon he was whistling along. When I stopped, he said, 'I enjoyed that. My wife can play the piano. She's got her ALCM.'

I was both stunned and distressed. How ever had he remembered the correct letters? But why, oh why, didn't he know that I was his wife?

The confusion continued. After our meal, I sat with him quietly and played one of his favourite records. He still couldn't say who I was. I showed him our wedding album and photos of the children when they were young. He actually named one or two people. But my name still escaped him and he looked at me as though he had never seen me before – even worse – as though he hated me!

I couldn't sleep. I was rehearsing all sorts of ways to remind him of who I was. Up until now, I had coped with everything that had happened. But here it was – the final straw. Perhaps I was getting it out of all proportion, common sense told me that I was. But I couldn't help it, I felt so hurt. How could he possibly forget who I was? Me, Audrey, his wife, the only person who had looked after him over all the years, the only one who knew how to cope, who knew about his strange little eccentricities. How could he forget me?

I was being silly and over-reacting. It was all part of the illness and something that I was going to have to accept. After all, people had told me that it was very often the person closest to them that they first forgot. But I hadn't really believed them – until now.

I lay there in the darkness feeling self-pity. For the first time in all the years of caring, I was thinking about myself and my life – all those wasted years, missed opportunities, never going anywhere, never doing anything – what a mess! Stan was sleeping peacefully. I buried my head in the pillow and continued to feel sorry for myself – but along with the sorrow was also the guilt. I was being stupid and selfish. It took a long time but gradually I became calmer. Things will be better tomorrow, I told myself as I drifted off to sleep.

Another day dawned – what sort of a day would it be? My day depended on Stan's day. I lay there quietly anticipating and hoping. I should really be up, taking the opportunity to get organised whilst Stan was still sleeping. I was still thinking about it when he began to stir.

Please, please let it be a good day – please let him know me!

My heart went out to him – he looked so young and healthy. No wonder that even now, after all these years, the rest of the world were still not prepared to accept that there was a problem.

He was awake and he looked straight at me and said, 'Hello love, is it morning?'

That was a wonderful start and my heart was racing. Please, please let it be true – I think my prayers have been answered. I think he knows me!

He gave me a lovely smile, snuggled down and closed his eyes again.

At breakfast he began to talk and he called me Audrey. I felt on top of the world. But, just as quickly, everything changed again.

'What's happening to me? Why can't I remember things?'

How could I answer such questions? I searched for the right words and finally convinced him that he was fine. Perhaps his memory was not very good but it didn't matter because I would remind him about things. And I would always be around to help him.

That reply seemed to satisfy him. But he upset me once more by saying, 'I am a mess. It's not fair for you. You don't deserve all this.'

Much later, he said, 'I haven't any money.' I reassured him by telling him that he had plenty of money and that I was looking after it for him. If he wanted any all he had to do was tell me.

'Oh, you are kind,' he said. 'My parents never give me any.'

19

Friday the Thirteenth

It was 1994 and it was May. I love this time of year when the gardens look so beautiful and the days are full of the promise of the summer still to come. The date was Friday the thirteenth!

I don't pretend to be superstitious but sometimes things happen and a little part of me will pinpoint something to which I attach more than a little significance. This time it was the date!

For quite some time, Stan had been spending less time at the Elgar Day Centre – a cost-cutting exercise was my guess – and instead, he had been going for one day a week to Timberdine Home, a lovely place not far from where we live.

My gut feeling about this was that, lovely though the place undoubtedly was, it really wasn't suitable for Stan, whose needs were becoming greater almost daily. The residents and day patients are well looked after and have lots of stimulation and lots of love. But (and what a big 'but' it turned out to be), they have to be able to blend in with the rest, to chatter and join in the activities. An impossibility for my poor darling. My doubts remained and my feeling was that the worse he was becoming, the less was the support that was being provided.

Anyway, back to Friday the thirteenth. Stan was collected as usual and I got ready to go into Worcester city to do the weekend shopping and keep a hair appointment. I was just ready to leave the house when the doorbell rang. It was Ann Barry from Timberdine – and Stan! It was 10.50.

'Whatever's the matter? Come in. What's wrong?' I was both concerned and surprised.

She came in. I took Stan's hand and we went through into the lounge.

'I'm sorry,' she said, 'we can't manage him any more.'

Before I could say anything, she went on, 'We tried to get him to settle but he was impossible. He wouldn't co-operate at all. He was shouting and being a nuisance and he was upsetting everybody.'

I looked at him, already seated in his usual chair, quite unconcerned and completely unaware of anything that was being said.

Ann continued. 'He was so noisy and disruptive – he wouldn't be quiet, he wouldn't sit down. None of the staff could manage him and the residents were frightened of him. It was awful.'

I glanced again at him, sitting there so quietly. He was no monster. He was my poor, confused and frightened husband. I could only guess what might have happened. Perhaps he had had one of his lucid moments – a sudden glimpse into what was happening. No wonder he was afraid and needed to make himself heard. No wonder he needed to rebel.

'We have to think of everyone else. We can't have them all upset. Rachel will be back on Monday and we'll talk things over then. And we'll be in touch with Keith.' (Rachel was the manager, who was on holiday.)

Ann was already walking towards the door, keen to make her escape.

'I'll be in touch.' And with that, she was gone. I knew with absolute certainty that Stan would never set foot in Timberdine again.

My mind was in a whirl. First came the practicalities. It would be Tuesday before Stan went to the Elgar Centre – five long days away. And I hadn't even started to do my 'Friday' things. I supposed we would get by, but I needed fresh food – vegetables, fruit, bread and my usual shopping for the weekend. My hair would have to go on looking a mess. I needed Fridays in so many ways. It was my breathing space and relaxation as I prepared myself for the physical and mental tiredness that the weekends always brought.

Then came my anger. They had obviously given no thought at all about my predicament. They couldn't manage – but somehow I had to, there was no alternative!

Monday came and went and I had heard nothing at all from either Timberdine or Keith at the Elgar Centre. On Tuesday morning, Stan went off to the Elgar Centre and when he had gone, I rang Keith to find out what was happening. He couldn't tell me anything and we seemed to have reached stalemate.

The last four days had been extremely long and tiring. Stan was going through one of his childhood phases. He pestered me to let him 'play out' because his mother said he could. He refused to let me shave him because razors were too dangerous to play with and he would have to 'go home' because he musn't be late for tea.

Late on Tuesday afternoon came the final ultimatum from Timberdine. It was as expected, there was no further place for Stan there. Then Keith rang. He had tried to find a place for him in West Wing but they were full.

So, in just five days, my world had been turned upside down, without warning and with complete disregard as to how I would manage. There would only be a few free hours on two days. The other five days Stan would be at home which meant that I too would be confined to the house. Getting about was now far too difficult for Stan; we had no car and public transport was impossible.

After 11 years of caring, everything had suddenly got on top of me. That most precious commodity, time, could not be properly used and it was being wasted.

The following day should have been a Timberdine day and, just to be perverse, Stan was lovely all day. He was quiet and seemed content. He was co-operative and the day passed without incident. But my timetable was up the creek. I had to cancel several appointments, I couldn't get down to the bank, a morning craft course came to a halt and I could no longer visit friends, as planned.

Just a final PS before I try to think of something more cheerful. I knew that Stan wasn't going to Timberdine on the Monday, so did the people in the home and at the Elgar Centre – but the transport still arrived to collect him. I couldn't help feeling bitter about that.

I'm getting to have quite a phobia about this timing business. Once again, things happened on the thirteenth and once again it was just days from his birthday!

105

Round about the same time, I had the distinct feeling that the doctor at the day centre was experimenting with Stan's medication and I became so concerned that I finally rang them and was able to speak to Dr Tarry. All she said was that if I was really concerned about him, I could give him another Haloperidol tablet. Early that same evening I was at my wit's end. I had had a full day of trying to cope with him. He had been argumentative and extremely aggressive. He had lashed out at me many times and I had been kicked and punched. He had also thrown a knife at me. Fortunately, it missed! But it impaled itself in one of the kitchen doors – the mark is still there. I had done as Dr Tarry suggested but the extra tablet hadn't made any difference – and I was fearful about giving him yet another one. So I had to ring our own doctor. It was Dr Solesbury who answered and she could hear Stan ranting and raving in the background. She told me to give him another and if he hadn't quietened down within half an hour she would come – it may mean getting him into hospital to be stabilised.

Thank goodness the extra tablet worked but never in my life had I felt so drained and exhausted.

The notes in my diary are so helpful and there are pages and pages of them. The last thing I want to be is boring – so I have decided to be selective. I will only write about events that, for one reason or another, I think will be of interest. Most of all, I want to make people understand (just a little bit) about what living with Alzheimer's is like.

Thursday, 17 November 1994 – Stan went to the Elgar Day Centre. At 3.45 the phone rang and it was Keith asking if Stan was home. I thought at the time it was strange but Keith explained that there had been a mix-up with the transport but I was not to worry.

4.30. I was getting very worried. Keith rang again and was very surprised when I told him there was still no sign of Stan.

4.45. Another call from Keith to assure me that all was well. I was not convinced, but Keith was reluctant to give me any more information.

5.15. Stan was nowhere to be seen. I rang the Elgar Centre. The phone was finally answered by a cleaning-lady – all the day care staff had left!

5.20. I got through to the ambulance station and asked them if they knew what was happening. They sounded very surprised but again told me not to worry.

5.25. I rang both Syd and Jim – I had to share my worries with somebody. They both came to the house. It must have looked like some sort of comedy act – the three of us, me in the middle, lined up at the front bedroom window of our bungalow and staring out into the darkness.

6.30. We had been stood there for over an hour. A car appeared out of the gloom. The driver got out and then helped Stan. What a relief! Whatever had happened?

Stan was my first priority. He was very agitated and absolutely desperate for the toilet. The driver (a new volunteer) had been given the wrong address and the wrong passenger. Because he was new, he never thought to find out whether Stan had his address on him – perhaps it would have been useless anyway. Stan never went anywhere without it, but the driver would have had to search through his pockets to find it. The driver also had no car phone – he finally managed to use a public call box and was told Aycliffe Road, Norton. Just Norton – not Norton Road, off the Bath Road in Worcester. The poor man had tried every Norton he could think of – and there are lots of them – he had even been out as far as Evesham and beyond. I felt so sorry for him – he really was upset and worried. He used the phone to contact his wife, refused my offer of a drink and left.

Stan had soon forgotten all about it. Once he was warm and had had something to eat he was fine. But just to add to my problems, during the night he tried to get up to go to the toilet. I got up straight away – but this time, I was too late. He just went down like a sack of potatoes and cracked his head on the corner of the wardrobe. He was covered in cuts and bruises on his arms and legs as well as his head.

Thursday 1 December – Stan was much worse and the day centre staff were very sympathetic. The doctor decided to keep him in West Wing to try to get him stabilised once more. I had got to the stage where I was just getting no sleep at all and they realised that I couldn't carry on like that with no extra help. I had my fingers crossed and hoped that something could be done to ease the situation.

Christmas 1994 – I would really rather forget all about it. It was an awful time. I had decided that it would be far better if Stan and I stayed here on our own. He wasn't fit to travel and I knew it would be too much for him if they all came here. I was also concerned about how I would cope – it was taking me all my time just to look after him.

I don't think I have ever felt quite so lonely and isolated. The only highlight was on Christmas Day when the family rang. Richard and Joy paid us a short visit after Christmas, before they set off on their usual trip to Scotland for the New Year. It was lovely to see them but also very exhausting. It made me realise just how tired I had become and how out of touch with normality. I still felt that Richard didn't realise just how time-consuming and demoralising looking after Stan was. Perhaps he did realise but was not yet prepared to accept there was a real problem.

In the New Year, Gillian and the family came over. It was another traumatic time for us all. At long last, they saw for themselves just a little bit of what I've had to deal with. I was upset by the aggression that Stan showed towards them but not surprised. Having to ring the doctor was another matter. I was thankful that Gillian was there – it helped a lot. At least they now knew some of my problems.

3 January 1995 – A different driver came to collect Stan to take him to the day centre. It was a lady and she parked the car in such a position that it was impossible for Stan to get into it. I asked her to move it so that I could help him – he always needed someone – but her response was to snap at us both.

'What's the matter with you, are you blind?' Little did she know that he was registered partially sighted, but at least she should have realised that he had Alzheimer's Disease.

'For goodness sake, hurry up. Just do what I tell you. You're just being stupid. Come on. Get a move on, you're making me late and I've got other people besides you.'

I finally managed to squeeze past the rose bushes, far too near where she had parked, and help Stan to get in. When they had gone, I cried and cried about her atrocious attitude. How could anyone be so cruel to someone so ill? She was so bad-tempered and lacking in understanding.

I simply had to report her – there was no way I could tolerate such treatment. 'Don't ever send her here again,' I insisted.

Just two days later, on the fifth, Stan's sister Doreen died. There was no point in saying anything at all to Stan. He would never comprehend what I was trying to say. Also on the very same day, the Elgar Day centre decided they had had enough. Stan would, in future, have to go to West Wing. Days later, whilst he was there, he had a fall and was very badly bruised. For the first time in all my years of caring, I then had a call from a health visitor whose advice was for me to look for a nursing home. We were getting close to another chapter in our lives.

Very soon, I am going to have to write about Stan finally having to go into a nursing home, but before then I want to let everyone know just how hard I fought throughout his illness to try to help him have some small degree of happiness for as long as possible. I have already written about going to Washington – I know that only happened because I had won a prize – but nevertheless it still took a lot of courage for me to decide to go.

So it has been throughout – but thanks to family and friends and such lovely neighbours, right up until his sixty-seventh birthday, the holidays and days out continued. They got more and more difficult as time went on, and quite honestly, a lot of the time, they weren't much fun for me – but I was determined to carry on.

Just to give you a taster, I will list some of them.

June 1987 – Eastbourne – that was the time when Stan got lost in the hotel. I found him in someone else's bedroom. Fortunately, they saw the funny side – they even realised there was a problem.

September – Saundersfoot, the first of many wonderful holidays with our neighbours, Peggy and Syd. We stayed in a luxury caravan on a superb site – they insisted it was going to be a real holiday for me – and I literally didn't have to lift a finger. They did allow Stan to wash up (it was the only thing he still tried to do). It took him forever, but they were so patient with him.

June 1988 – Jersey. A chapter of accidents for me – I broke a window in the hotel and broke my glasses. But it was lovely to see Stan relaxing in the sunshine.

August – Rhine valley. We only managed this because we were with our friends, Fay and Mike. The biggest mishap was losing Stan on the boat.

April 1989 – Brecon Beacons with Richard and Joy – we stayed in a guest house and Stan was fine. Richard and Joy went off on their own.

March 1991 – Norfolk Broads and Norwich. Again with Richard and Joy.

August – Saundersfoot again. This time with Gillian and family. We lost Stan on Barafundle beach.

April 1992 – Symonds Yat. Again we were with Richard and Joy and again we lost Stan.

That is just a sample of what all those lovely people were doing to try and help us. I really don't know how I would have managed without them. But for things like that to look forward to, I am certain I would not have managed half as well.

Anyway, back to the Christmas of 1994 and the beginning of 1995. Stan still continued to be very unwell and was giving me cause to worry about him even more than usual. Round about the middle of January, the Elgar Centre finally transferred Stan into West Wing. I didn't like the idea and told them so – they then dangled a carrot in front of me and said he could go there on Sundays as well as the other two days. Dr Solesbury also called to see me and said she would try to arrange for me to have some help at home. At last, I thought that help was on the way. But then Stan started having a lot of pain and a community nurse visited him to try and make him more comfortable. Her visits continued until the middle of February, when he went for yet another stay in West Wing.

I took the opportunity to look at nursing homes whilst he was in respite care. Another friend, Sonia, went with me and I finally chose Welland House, a lovely old house close to the Malvern Hills. They normally had a long waiting list, but for once I had chosen the right time – they had just completed a brand new extension with extra bedrooms, some of which were still available. I took the plunge and said that I would like Stan to go there. He would be able to have one of the new bedrooms, complete with its own bathroom facilities. Everything in the room would be brand new. I was introduced to the staff that were on duty – all very caring and understanding, and all very friendly. The senior staff were all trained in the care of mental health patients.

At the weekend, Gillian and family arrived. They wanted to see for themselves and they agreed with me that it seemed ideal. I knew it wouldn't be long before I would have to let Stan go. It was on my mind all day and all night, and I was full of so many conflicting emotions about it.

As it happened, the final decision was beyond my control – it was taken right out of my hands.

20

Extra-Curricular Activities

At the same time as we were journeying through this most awful of all nightmares and I was watching in helpless dismay the deterioration of my wonderful husband, I began to get involved in what I can only describe as extra-curricular activities. I suppose there were two main reasons for my involvement, the first one being to spread the word about Alzheimer's Disease – which was still a total mystery to so many people, including some of the professionals. My second reason was a more selfish one. For so many years I had kept all the anxieties and problems close to my heart, not wanting to admit, even to myself, that there was a problem. Now, by beginning to open up and talk to others about our experiences, I found it was acting as some sort of therapy for me. Instead of always bottling things up, I began to relax.

The first thing I would like to tell you about was our decision to take part in some drug trials. I read an article about these trials in *The Times* and casually mentioned them to Stan. I didn't really expect any reaction and was therefore amazed when he almost jumped down my throat and said, 'Well, that's it then. What are we waiting for?' He was grasping at straws, I knew that. But he wanted to do something, anything, that might help, and I found myself contacting the Institute of Psychiatry, at the Maudsley Hospital in London. Their reply came in March 1989, inviting us to attend an interview on May the thirty-first, which would last from 9.30 a.m. until about 3.00 p.m.

The only way we could be there for that time was by staying overnight at Gillian's and then getting a train to Waterloo. I discussed everything with Gillian and she was keen for us to try – she would also like to come with us to the hospital. And so it was all arranged. We were introduced to Professor Raymond Levy and the nature of the trials and our involvement was all explained. The drug being tested was a choline esterase inhibitor, tetrahydro-aminoacridine, shortened to THA, which would be combined with lecithin. The patients must have uncomplicated forms of the disease. The risk of liver damage was explained, the carer had to take responsibility for administering the medication exactly as prescribed and be prepared to arrange fortnightly visits to the hospital for monitoring and assessment.

Gillian was more than ready to offer overnight stays for us so that we would be able to keep all the appointments. Professor Levy was keen for Stan to take part and so it was all settled.

The trials lasted for two years and altogether we made 31 visits to the hospital. These were obviously all at our own expense – but I didn't count the cost of that. The benefits far outweighed the costs – it kept us in touch with Gillian, it gave both of us some-thing to look forward to, it kept Stan's hopes high and perhaps some good might just come out of all the research.

I was very interested in the tests that they were using – in fact, they used me as a guinea pig, I even had to have the blood tests. Going down on the train, Stan would sometimes remember that they would be asking him some questions and he would ask me to test him. I knew he wouldn't remember the answers and so we often played that game to pass the time.

He needed to be able to tell them his name, address and age – to know what day it was and what time, month, season and year. He also needed to tell them just where he was – what sort of place, what floor, what town. He was asked basic things such as the name of the Prime Minister, date of World Wars One and Two. He had to recognise pictures of everyday objects, reproduce very basic shapes and count backwards from 20. As the visits continued his scoring rate gradually decreased and he began to get rather irri-tated and restless. Unfortunately, the tests came to nothing – but we had the satisfaction of knowing that at least we had tried.

Another thing I did was to join a carers' group organised by Caroline Sincock, the clinical psychologist at the hospital where

Stan went for day care. In fact, I was one of the founder members. I was instrumental in starting a carers' magazine for them and have contributed a number of articles for them (see Afterword). I also wrote articles for the Alzheimer's Disease Society and a poem written when Stan was still at home, which appeared in several local publications.

In 1992, I was asked to go and talk to some trainee nurses at the local hospital who were starting a course on mental health. It was an introduction to a much bigger event held at our local theatre. It was a full-day conference attended by delegates from all over the area involved in the care of the elderly and/or the mentally ill. I found myself in the company of all manner of distinguished people who had come along to speak at this event. My talk was scheduled for after lunch, so I had plenty of time to get thoroughly nervous and wonder what on earth I was doing there. I suppose my teacher training came to the rescue – within seconds of starting, I found my nervousness disappearing. I knew exactly what I wanted to say and I also felt that the audience were very receptive. I had my poem with me, but wasn't sure beforehand whether or not it would be right for this occasion. I threw caution to the winds and finished my talk by reading it out to them. I now know what the expression 'you could have heard a pin drop' really means. I got to the end of my poem – there was complete and utter silence! Then came the applause. It was loud and it was long, and I actually saw people (some of them men) dabbing their eyes.

Who Am I? – I Think, Therefore I Am!

I think. Oh yes, I think – of what and why and how?
    The thoughts go tumbling through my brain
    I look for solace. I find the pain –
Of thinking of the life we had – and what that life is now.

I think of all the plans we had for spending life together.
    Our partnership was oh so good,
    Sharing everything – as we should.
The thoughts I have at night are worst. The nights go on forever.

114

I think about the days gone by – our happiness together.
>Our optimism and our plans
>To face the future, hand-in-hand.
Confident and full of hope that joy would last forever.

We are together even now – but in such a different way.
>Vague memories he still retains
>Confusing thoughts torment his brain.
Together still – but *I'm* alone, to face life day by day.

I think of *his* emotions. What feelings has he still?
>Dulled in his whole approach to life.
>How can I help him, as his wife?
I'm wife *and* mother to him now – all duties to fulfil.

I think of *my* emotions – all my loneliness and fears.
>Will I manage? Will I cope?
>Guilt feelings, feelings of losing hope,
I think of all my tiredness, as days drag into years.

I think about the present, but don't like what I think.
>Help with shaving, washing, dressing,
>All life's trivia – so depressing!
Then I see his look of thanks – my eyes fill to the brink.

I think of what is said to me. 'Try to lead a normal life.'
>I try so hard – I really do.
>But I'm so tired – so much to do.
And all I really want has gone. Our life together – man and wife.

I think about the future. What else has life in store?
>Long years of caring without cease.
>Sometimes, I wish for his release –
But how will I continue – each day, I love him more.

It's not the love of early days – those heady days of yore.
>But love that deepens with the years
>Compassion, overflowing tears,
Heartache for the man he is, grief for what he was before.

115

I think. Oh yes I think – of how, and what and why?
>I pray for strength to carry on
>As many, many more have done.
I pray for sleep. I pray for rest. I pray that I won't cry.

It had all been so worthwhile. A collection was held and £300 donated to the Alzheimer's Disease Society. A few days later, I received a lovely letter of thanks from the person who had organised the event, with the very true comment, 'we can all walk away at the end of our day – you can't'. Then came the flowers and the cards – and an article in the local paper.

I suppose it was because of that talk that I was approached by local radio to speak about Alzheimer's. I called myself 'Jean' – it fooled some of the people but I still got calls about it from those who had recognised my voice. And I found myself being contacted for advice from other worried carers.

Sometime later, I completed a form from the BBC. It was an *Age Watch* survey about a future programme that they were hoping to make. I almost didn't send it off as some of the questions were rather vague and many didn't have enough space for the full-page reply that the question warranted. But eventually I completed it, sent it off and forgot all about it. It was months later when I had a phone call from a BBC producer who wanted to come and see us both. I resisted in vain – gradually I was won over, with the result that I finally agreed to them filming us for a documentary about retirement entitled 'Never Too Late'. Our contribution was about the downside.

I don't intend to go into the details about filming, which took two days, except to say what exciting but exhausting days they were. I rang Gillian once everyone had left. I knew she would want to know all about it. I gave her as full an account as I could and she wanted to know how her dad had been.

'He's here, stood right beside me. I'll let him tell you about it.' I handed the phone over to him and Gillian repeated her question. We neither of us could believe his reply.

'No, nothing happened. It was just an ordinary day.'

But he was the only one who thought like that. After the broadcast, we were inundated with letters, cards, phone calls and per-

116

sonal callers to the house. Then came one important call from the Alzheimer's Disease Society. Would I possibly help with the making of a video? Just where was it all going to end?

Michael Barrett was the producer this time and the routine was now familiar. The whole recording took just two hours and the 30-minute video *Looking at Alzheimer's Disease* is now readily available. I have a personal copy of an unedited version of the same thing which is very precious to me. Stan tried so valiantly to find the right words. He obviously thought he was back at work and expressed the hope that 'his staff had shown them the whole system.' He thanked them for their visit, which he described as 'immaculate' and he referred to our marriage as 'fruitful'. Not quite the right words but if this video helps to provide more understanding and ways of coping, then perhaps 'fruitful' is a good word to use, after all.

It wasn't long after the making of this video that things came to a head and Stan had to be admitted to hospital – and from there to a nursing home. I now found myself with time on my hands – the first time for many years. I decided to rejoin the local Alzheimer's group, which for many years I had been unable to attend.

Never one to do anything by halves, I was, in one fell swoop, invited to join the committee and, as though that wasn't enough, I became their new treasurer. And just to make sure that I was doing all I could, I was also invited to become a carers' contact for the region. So I still don't have very much spare time!

My work in all these areas has helped me enormously to come to terms with our situation. I have met so many other carers, directly through the local groups and indirectly through the many moving articles and books written by them. I, myself, have been contacted on several occasions by the Alzheimer's Disease Society in London with a variety of requests from them – for me to write something for their monthly newsletter, review a book, talk to the media, and help in many other ways. It has made me realise that I am just one of many, all with the same problems, fears, grief and the never-ending tiredness that accompanies all the care. Many of the things that have been written have reduced me to tears and my heart has gone out to everyone. Some of the expressions that have been used are so very poignant and meaningful.

Some of the ways of coping with difficult situations have struck home and many of the solutions to problems have been very helpful to me.

For a long time, one of my major problems was 'losing' him. I have already mentioned it in passing, and in retrospect, it all now sounds rather amusing – but it certainly wasn't amusing at the time. One of the articles I sent to the Alzheimer's Disease Society was entitled 'I Love to Go a-Wandering'. Perhaps I can quote from this:

We loved it, the Yorkshire Dales, the Lake District when we were in the North, and here in the Midlands, the Malverns, the Cotswolds and the beautiful river valleys. Walking was still 'the tops'. But things changed with Stan's illness – and he began to wander. Escape from the house came first and then the real wandering began.

I lost him in all sorts of peculiar places. Actually, Jeremy – our son-in-law – lost him first. We were staying in Berkshire and the two of them, plus the dog, had gone for a walk. Jeremy popped into the local garage. When he came out, both Stan and the dog had completely vanished. It was in a thickly wooded area with paths in all directions and – to cut a long story short – a full search party had to be launched. Several hours later, they were both finally spotted by the police, close to the M4 motorway and miles away from our daughter's house. Peter, the dog, was so exhausted he never left his basket all the rest of the night or the following day.

Shops were a nightmare! They were soon on the 'not to be recommended' list. One glance into a shop window, one moment's lapse of attention and he would be gone!

An amazing escape happened in the Wye Valley where we had gone with Richard and Joy. The two of them had gone off on their own at Symonds Yat, leaving us relaxing on a seat about halfway up the hill between river and road. Stan got a bit restless and started walking up and down and then back to the seat again. He didn't go out of sight so I was quite happy. Again, it only took a matter of seconds and he was gone – out of sight round a corner. But which corner? Did I go to look for him up or down the hill? I did both to no avail. By the time Richard and Joy came back, I was frantic. We looked everywhere and finally got back in the car and drove slowly along the main road. It was the last resort. All at once, Richard spotted him. He was in a phone box!

I still can't credit it – but here was this man who no longer answered the phone and had certainly never made a phone call himself for years – actually using a public telephone. He had realised he was lost and had dialled 999 and was actually talking to the police when Richard spotted him! Thank goodness the policeman had detected from Stan's voice that there was a problem and was keeping him talking whilst a police car had been sent out to look for him.

On another occasion, we were away in South Wales with Gillian and the family and thoroughly enjoying a gorgeous sunny day on one of our favourite beaches – Barafundle. The two boys were exploring some caves, Gillian and I were in the sea and Jeremy and Stan were sunbathing on the beach. Suddenly, Jeremy gave an enormous shout and went hell for leather up the steep steps to the cliff top. He was just in time to catch up with Stan before he set off on the Pembrokeshire Way footpath. Again, nobody had seen him go and he was climbing the path like a mountain goat. Who would ever believe that this was the same person we almost gave up on? We none of us thought he would make it down to the beach!

When we asked him what he thought he was doing, his reply was 'I was just taking some photographs' … without a camera?!!

Railway stations held a strange attraction for him. The place – Reading station, platform four. The train for Worcester was due at any minute, it was already signalled. Gillian, Jeremy and the boys had come to see us off and we were all waiting together. That's what we thought!

'Grandma,' said Simon, 'look at Grandad walking over the bridge!' This was the man who found steps difficult, refused to use escalators and seconds earlier had been stood with us. How we got him back and caught the train, I'll never know!

My worst nightmare was at another railway station. This

time it was Liverpool Street Station in the rush hour. I was juggling with the luggage and scanning the indicator board to find the platform we needed. Stan was stood by my side. But, suddenly, he wasn't! He had been swept along with the crowd and vanished into thin air. I panicked! What if he had got on a train – any train, going who knows where? It was the worst few moments of my life. How I spotted him I'll never know and how I managed to calm down and take control of things again is another of life's mysteries. Ironically, the platform we needed was number 13!

So he did wander – and I did lose him. But at the end of the last chapter I mentioned that he finally had to go into a nursing home. Somehow, I have got to pluck up the courage to write about that – I can't leave it for much longer. I have to write about the biggest loss of all!

21

The Nursing Home

My heart is so heavy but I have got to bring myself to write about the events of early 1995. Only a few weeks, but the longest few weeks of my life. Our doctor, as promised, had arranged for a bath nurse to come once a week. That lightened the load for me and I just 'topped and tailed' him as best I could on the other days. Thank goodness he was still continent. I feel that was mainly because of my vigilance rather than his understanding. The bath nurse was the only help I received. How I would have welcomed a little bit more.

Stan's deterioration had accelerated and it was heartbreaking to see him. He was having more and more falls. In fact, he had fallen in West Wing just before Michael Barrett did his filming. His face was covered in bruises but the film crew had been able to concentrate on his good side for most of the time.

We somehow struggled through January but in early February Stan collapsed three times in the space of a week. The first time it happened, the ambulance men had just arrived to take him to day care. They were so good with him and brought him round. In West Wing, he was examined by the doctor and the staff kept an eye on him all day. He seemed to be OK. But the next day, he had another funny turn, which didn't last long but made me worried. When it happened for a third time, just a couple of days later, it seemed worse and I contacted our doctor.

He was over it by the time Dr Solesbury arrived but she arranged for him to go into Ronkswood Hospital straight away for tests. It was already late in the evening and by the time the tests were all completed, it was one o'clock the following day. They weren't admitting him and so I had to find transport and get him back home.

The following day was a Saturday. Stan looked so tired and ill and was refusing to eat anything. I felt helpless just watching him. By Sunday he was worse and I was extremely worried. I contacted our doctor yet again. Dr Deighton, one of the doctors I had never met before, arrived at lunchtime. His first words when he saw Stan were, 'You have a very sick man here.' He gave him a thorough examination and then said, 'We must get him into hospital straight away.'

My emotions were so mixed – an overwhelming sadness to see Stan like this, but also relief that at long last somebody was taking notice of what I had been saying for a week.

Stan was placed in a single room in Ward 2, Newtown Hospital. It was my first experience of hospital care. I do wish I could give a glowing report but, in reality, it was an awful experience. I had given them the full details which they required and everything had been written down. They referred to him as 'John'. I explained that John was one of his names, but he had always been called Stan. On my next visit, his name was displayed above his bed – JOHN – in large letters. I asked them to change it. They didn't. Finally, I had to change it myself. I explained that he couldn't feed himself or even manage a drink without help. I also told them he was partially sighted and couldn't see the food on his plate or the drink in his beaker. On my next visit, I found a full cup of tea, untouched and stone-cold, and a complete meal of meat and vegetables, all congealed and unappetising – and again untouched. The cutlery hadn't been used at all. It had obviously been placed there and, in spite of the information I had given them, he was expected to get on and feed himself. His lips looked dry and cracked and his eyes were caked and looked very sore.

I asked a nurse what was going on. She just shrugged her shoulders and said, 'I'll find out for you.' I never saw her again.

Every visit was the same. More often than not, Syd came with me. Once again he was wonderful. He was just as concerned as I was about the care Stan was getting. Stan's appearance was becoming more and more unkempt – he was often unshaven and his hair looked all matted and tangled.

I asked about his treatment and the only response I got was, 'We are doing some tests' – that's all I ever got to know and his chart did nothing to enlighten me.

Oh what a place! I couldn't wait to get him out of there – and this is where things were taken out of my hands. It was agreed that, when Stan was well enough to leave the hospital, it would be best for everyone if he was transferred straight away to Welland House.

I expect you are able to guess by now that when the actual date for transferring Stan was fixed it could only be one date – the thirteenth!

Arrangements were made for the ambulance to bring him over. Gillian, bless her, came over to Worcester on the twelfth of March. I was so glad that she could be with me. I know I couldn't have coped on my own. We arrived at Welland before the ambulance was due and we were talking to Maureen (the nurse in charge) in her office. She was filling in all the details she needed to know about Stan. She had just asked if he was still continent and I was so pleased to be able to say 'Yes'. It was then that the ambulance arrived and Gillian and I went to meet it. The first thing we both noticed was the smell – he had soiled himself! What a start! Maureen was sympathetic. She made no fuss, simply asked a nurse to 'make him comfortable'. They took over, quietly and calmly, and we were then able to introduce him to Maureen and some of the other staff.

There are no words to describe how I felt – there was sadness, numbness and shock – but there was also relief. A guilty sort of relief at this point in time – but already I had begun to realise that the burden of caring was no longer weighing so heavily on my shoulders.

I prayed that I had made the right decision and that Stan would continue to get the tender loving care that he deserved.

I had entered a new phase of my life and was finding it so very strange. Time, that elusive commodity, was now on my side again – but I didn't know what to do with it. I still found myself awake very early and unable to settle again. I still planned a timetable when really there was no longer any need. Gradually, as the days passed, I found the fatigue which I had felt for so many years was beginning to disappear.

But my emotions were another matter. I knew Stan was receiving the best of all possible care. I knew he didn't realise where he was and why he was there. I knew it had been the only possible solution – but I still felt so guilty and distressed by my failure to keep my promise. I could still hear his words – 'You'll never leave me, will you?' and my reply – 'I'll always be here to take care of you.'

I couldn't get to Welland House without help – public transport was non-existent – but I had thought long and hard about that before I made my decision. The nursing home were fully aware of how 'out in the sticks' they were. They were fully prepared to help out with transport. Bill, their odd-job man and driver, has come to my rescue on many occasions – it has never been any problem. But again, it was the wonderful neighbours who have (and still do) stick by me and take it in turns to take me over there.

'We think the world of Stan. He's still our friend and we want to see him just as much as you do.' What wonderful neighbours they are!

At the beginning, Stan wasn't too well – he arrived at Welland with a urinary infection and a foot infection, cellulitis. Two weeks after he arrived, they still hadn't had any information about him from Newtown Hospital. We were all disgusted but I couldn't say I was surprised. I was also waiting for them to find his electric razor, which had gone missing. I was horrified to think that it had possibly been used to shave another patient. Gillian and Richard managed to come over and see their dad. They did their utmost to assure me that I had done the right thing. I was slowly beginning to think that they were right.

The third of June was our forty-fifth wedding anniversary and Enid and Harry (our bridesmaid and best man) came over from Bristol. They were shocked to see Stan. I had tried to warn them but they were still unprepared for the change in him. He was going through a period of aggression and was being restrained in his chair, for his own safety as well as the safety of everyone else. I had planned to have a holiday in Italy with Richard and Joy. The staff begged me not to change my plans and insisted it was just a passing phase.

The holiday was wonderful – beautiful Lake Garda, the Dolomites on probably the very best day of the year, Venice on another gorgeous day – I came back refreshed and happy, only to find that Stan was still disturbed. His behaviour was noisy and aggressive and they were having to sedate him, which they never liked to do.

Gillian and the boys came over again for the August Bank Holiday. After seeing Stan, who was remarkably bright and cheerful, we took advantage of the weather and had a lovely walk on the Malverns. How Stan would have enjoyed it! The phone was ringing as we arrived home – it was Steve from Welland House with the news that Stan had fallen and broken his hip. They were waiting for the ambulance to take him to hospital. I wanted to go to the hospital to be with him but Steve insisted that I stayed away. 'It's my job – it's likely to take a very long time to get everything sorted. I shall stay with him, however long it takes. Shall I ring you when I know something or shall I leave it until tomorrow morning?' He was adamant and there was no point in arguing – it was sensible, too. I couldn't do anything if I was there. But I insisted he ring me straight away. I couldn't wait until the morning. Gillian and the boys should have been going back to Bracknell the following day but rang Jeremy to say they would stay here until they knew what was going to happen.

It was well after midnight when Steve rang. Stan's hip was broken and he had been transferred to Worcester Royal Infirmary. Steve was just waiting to see him settled and then he would be going home. The date was the second of August.

It was three days later, on the fifth, before the operation was carried out. The operation should have been on the third – it was cancelled because of an emergency. It was cancelled again on the fourth – another emergency. I tried in vain to follow the logic – what was Stan's predicament? Surely that was also an emergency?

When the operation was finally carried out – it was a full hip replacement – Stan was fine and Gillian was able to go back home. The staff on the ward were marvellous – they knew about Stan's dementia but it made no difference. They took on board the extra care and said, 'We love him.' What a difference to his treatment in Newtown.

The one thing that did upset me was being informed by a 'friend' that when other 'friends' were talking about what had happened, including the delay in operating, they had simply said, 'Well, they have to deal with emergencies first, and it doesn't really matter about someone like him. And what about all those on a waiting list?'

I couldn't believe it! What was Stan if not an emergency? And what have waiting lists got to do with it? How unthinking can people be?

I discovered later that Stan's fall was caused by another resident charging into him and knocking him over. The man died very soon afterwards.

It had really knocked the stuffing out of Stan. He was very thin and gaunt and I could never get any response from him. He was always sleepy and he wasn't eating. Two months later, Maureen was very concerned. 'We are just watching him fade away.' I felt she was warning me about what may happen.

It was the beginning of October before Stan started to eat again. He still wasn't standing, let alone trying to walk.

Friday the thirteenth – well it simply had to be that date, didn't it? It was still October and it was the start of yet another awful time. Richard had come over to give a talk at his old grammar school – it was their careers evening. He had been invited on several occasions and always thoroughly enjoyed speaking. This time Joy was with him but I felt a strange tension between them that I really couldn't define. We had arranged to visit Stan the following day. I knew Richard would be upset but he was absolutely heartbroken and had to go out of the room in order to compose himself. It turned out to be more than his dad who was upsetting him. On the way back from the nursing home, he and Joy had a blazing row and straight after she had had her lunch, Joy left without a thank-you or a backward glance. Poor Richard was devastated but not prepared to unburden himself. He left early on Sunday morning – I felt certain we had both had a sleepless night.

That was the last I saw of Joy. Both she and Richard were find-

126

ing that they were growing apart and, strong characters that they both undoubtedly were, neither would give way. They had already reached the stage when the differences between them would not be reconciled. The split was inevitable. I felt completely drained. I couldn't bear to see Richard looking so upset. As though I hadn't enough to worry about!

The rest of 1995 dragged on with very little to cheer about. More often than not, Stan didn't know me – the only red-letter days were when he gave me a smile. For most of that time he was being extremely noisy and disruptive. Maureen spoke to me again about his quality of life and the fact that they were having to sedate him.

I have very little recorded in my diary for 1996. Stan's walking was very spasmodic. There were days when he wouldn't walk at all and others when he was on the go all day long. March the thirteenth (exactly one year since he went to Welland) passed without incident.

My next entry was on the day before he was 70. He had had another accident. Bernard, another resident who was extremely unsteady, collided with him with the result that Stan's head went straight through a plate-glass window. The staff were very concerned indeed – they had been unable to reach the two of them in time to prevent the collision. It could have been an absolute disaster. Stan was badly cut around his eyes and there was extensive bruising – thank goodness that was where it ended.

Monday the twentieth of May was Stan's 70th birthday. Syd took me over to see him and we tried to make the day a bit special with a cake for everyone to share and lots of cards and presents for Stan. I hope he knew it was something special but there was no way of really knowing. His face, after the accident the previous day, was awful and he was unable to open his left eye.

A month later, he had his third accident. This time he trapped three fingers in a door. Once again he didn't seem to be aware of what had happened.

As 1996 drew to a close, it was also another of Stan's noisy times. Each time I visited him, I could hear him long before I got into the main room. It must be dreadful for the staff to have to cope – he is just one of many, all with dementia and all causing

127

problems. I felt relieved for them once the noisy stage subsided, which was many, many weeks later.

But then I felt I had something else to worry about. There had been more falls, more bruising until, once again, Stan decided he wasn't going to walk any more. He went completely rigid every time anyone tried to get him to stand up. That meant a wheelchair whenever he needed to go anywhere. Otherwise, thank goodness, he was beginning to look better and was once more eating and sleeping well.

22

Not Just the Old

My story is drawing to a close. The details I have chosen to write about are just a few picked out more or less at random from so many others – just a glimpse of what it is like.

Quite recently, I attended a one-day conference and the speaker's subject was 'The Younger Person with Dementia'. As I listened, I thought that's us – he's telling our story and probably making a better job of it than I ever could.

He was putting forward a very strong case for the recognition of the fact that Alzheimer's Disease is not just a disease of old age. And, even more importantly, that younger sufferers and their carers have very different problems and needs.

Statistics show that as many as one person in five over the age of 80 may be showing signs of dementia, ranging from mild to severe. Between the ages of 65 and 70, only about two people in a hundred will show any signs, and below that age – from 40 to 65 – there may be perhaps one person out of a thousand with signs of Alzheimer's Disease. A very small number – but such people have very different problems that should be taken very seriously and looked at in detail.

A small number it may be, but when one of that number happens to be someone very close to you, then everything he spoke about had special significance for me. Stan was most certainly one of those statistics.

Here are just some of the points he raised that I would like to comment upon.

1. The younger person may still be physically fit. Stan certainly was, hence his need to continue walking for as long as possible. When he was at home, I got him out as much as possible – but at the day centre, full of very elderly people, Stan was immediately the odd one out. His wandering about was probably a nuisance. It was much easier for the staff to have everyone sitting quietly, probably dozing, or possibly exercising gently whilst still seated. Not really the right sort of care for a still active younger person.

2. A younger person often has more awareness of what is happening. That was my main reason for taking part in research on THA. I obviously hoped it would prove to be some sort of breakthrough – but my main reason was that Stan himself insisted on taking part. He knew all too well what was happening to him. That was so heartbreaking for me and so difficult to cope with.

3. The younger person still retains his special character. Stan certainly still had a very strong character. He hadn't sunk into that 'limbo' peculiar to older people – he was the same Stan as always, with his own individual sense of humour and sense of propriety. He still wanted to be part of the action.

Those are just some of the physical, psychological and personality differences between someone like Stan, still in his fifties and sixties, to the rest – all 70 plus, and many in their eighties and nineties.

The points made by the speaker, a specialist in the care of Alzheimer's patients, were so valid. There really should be separate facilities, more clinical investigation, more counselling (in our case, that was nil) and much more recognition of the needs of both the younger patient and the carer.

I simply don't understand why it appears to be so difficult for the different services to get their act together and look into the needs of the younger sufferer. In all my time of caring, we never once had a visit from a social worker, health visitor, community nurse or anyone from the voluntary sector. The closest we ever got to any 'help' was a bath nurse, once a week, when Stan was almost 69 and only weeks away from going into a nursing home, and someone from the council discussing finance with respect to the nursing home fees. How I would have welcomed help at a much earlier stage, which could have meant I would have been able to care for Stan for longer!

But, over and above all the physical and psychological 'mishandling' by those in charge – and the gradual deterioration that I had to cope with because there was simply no alternative – there were so many other problems, financial and social, which were much harder to sort out.

First came the loss of active and paid employment, not just for Stan, but very soon for me as well. Imagine the shock of suddenly being thrown onto the scrap heap at 55. No longer would there be a substantial salary at the end of each month – but our expenses would remain the same, there would be no diminution here. When I, too, had to finish work, it was doubly hard. My ambition to teach had come late and then disappeared far too early.

Life as a carer was a labour of love. There was no state recognition of my role and no pay. But again, we survived – living on Invalidity Benefit and very depleted company pensions. Our son was part-way through his university course. We managed to see him achieve his ambition. Not only that, we then helped him through a second degree course, essential for his career. I was determined that children and grandchildren should never have to suffer through our misfortunes. Thank goodness we had been prudent – something we learned through our knowledge of the hardships that both sets of parents had had to face.

Benefits such as Invalid Care Allowance were not for us. They didn't exist when we needed them – and by the time they did exist, I was too old to claim anything. Stubbornness, pig-headedness, or maybe just pure ignorance also meant a long delay before we received Attendance Allowance and longer still to get the Mobility Allowance.

So much for the financial side. But it was the rapid social isolation that was the most difficult of all. Fortunately, our true friends stayed with us, but there was a steady decline in the number of people who called to see us, to ring up just for a chat or to suggest outings. Even worse, I was aware that some people were actually avoiding us, when we were outside. I pretended that it didn't hurt – but inside there was a voice shouting, 'It's not catching. We are still people and we still have feelings!'

There was so much need for counselling for us and education for the rest of society.

That need is still there. Why can't there be more co-operation between health, social and voluntary services? Why can't there be consultants, doctors and social workers with special responsibility for the care of younger people with dementia? Why can't there be special training for recognising the symptoms of early onset dementia? Why can't there then be proper provision for the on-going supervision of these younger patients? All the specialist services should also be readily available and (more importantly) suitable for the differing needs of younger people with dementia and their carers.

And finally, if employers could be educated and informed about early onset dementia, perhaps it might lead to a positive response from them. If they could be made to realise that early onset dementia may lead to early and permanent retirement, then they may be persuaded to arrange a special pension with built-in rights and other benefits.

And so to my final chapter – all I have written so far has been a true account of life with Alzheimer's Disease. Try if you can to think of some of these events. Multiply everything by anything up to 20 times a day, 7 days and nights a week, 52 weeks a year and for at least 12 years (a very conservative estimate). That will give you a clearer picture of what looking after someone with this awful disease is really like. Every day and night brought so many problems and with them, the sheer exhaustion of never being able to relax.

For my final chapter I am trying hard to think of something happy and positive – what better than St Valentine's Day 1997 – and that is where my story will end.

23

Memories

February the fourteenth 1997 – St Valentine's Day. In the post amongst all the usual boring correspondence was an envelope, larger and more colourful than all the rest. It was a valentine card from Stan. It was so unexpected and so lovely that I simply dissolved into tears. I hugged it and kissed it and held it close to me whilst feeling both happy and sad at the same time. Someone had helped him to write his name in very spidery letters. Someone had obviously thought about making my day special and I was thrilled.

I thought back to the valentine card I had had many years previously. It was another precious card that Stan had made at the day centre. I still have it carefully stored away with all my souvenirs. It was folded – not quite straight – down the centre. It had a lurid red heart and the inevitable gold arrow. The card was too well drawn to be Stan's work but I like to think some of it was done by him. Perhaps the pink ribbon had been stuck on by him – it was crooked and blobs of glue stained the surface. The message inside was the same as always – 'With all my love' – someone else had written it but he had written his name, with a great deal of help, of that I am certain. It was a perfect card, in spite of all its imperfections.

And now, in 1997, here I was with another one! It is the little things like this that have helped me to cope throughout all the years of caring. All I have left are memories of the fleeting moments of togetherness – the smiles I have had, the words he has managed to say that have meant 'thank you' and the looks that have meant 'thank you' when no words would come. I cling to those memories.

I remember the laughter too – there was lots of it. It could have been tears of frustration when I found the bag full of rubbish in the fridge instead of in the dustbin. But we laughed – both of us – and it was so therapeutic. We laughed when Stan went to get a sweater from the bedroom and came back into the lounge draped in his duvet. And there were lots of smiles when he sang along to the piano as I played some of the old tunes. There was more laughter when he put the wrong words (rather naughty words) to some of them.

There has also been the satisfaction of a job well done – from the everyday things like washing, dressing, shaving, toileting, eating and drinking. It only took a smile from Stan as I helped him, and the rest of the day would be fine. And, as for the bigger things – days out, holidays, visits to London and America – they were all so worthwhile. They took a lot of planning and a lot of courage, but I am now so thankful that we did all of them. There are so many happy memories for me and, who knows, maybe even an occasional glimpse of something for Stan. That's probably wishful thinking but I can go on dreaming, can't I?

There could have been so much bitterness. There have been so many broken dreams and unfulfilled ambitions. Timing has never been on our side. In the early days, when we did have time, we didn't have the money. Then it was time to take care of careers and children that got in the way. And now, for over a quarter of our married life, my time has been spent in watching Stan grow steadily worse and trying to cope with so many sticky problems. Time has never been on my side, whilst time for Stan is meaningless.

I am aware that for many years I have been living a sort of bereavement but I have no idea at all about how I will cope with a real one. Everything that lies ahead is unknown and all I can do is what I have been doing for so many years – live a day at a time and fill every minute as usefully and pleasantly as I can. I cannot help my emotions – bitterness, despair, anger, remorse, guilt, self-pity. They are the awful, negative ones. But there must be room for happy thoughts – I try to brush aside the sadness and think of making every moment as happy as possible.

If yesterday was happy, then today can have happy thoughts

and tomorrow I will remember only the happiness. It's a hard philosophy to live by and I know there are still many hurdles to overcome. But I am convinced that with just a little bit more determination, I will succeed and this matter of timing will no longer be the enemy that has always been there. Time will no longer count – it will be just a commodity to be used to the full.

Like time, my story hasn't really got an end. All I hope is that it will be treated kindly by all those fortunate people untouched by Alzheimer's who will perhaps now have just a glimmer of what it is like. I hope it will help them to look with more compassion and understanding at sufferers, like Stan and their carers, like myself – who have made or are still making that same journey.

One day, the word 'Alzheimer's' will be known and understood by everyone. It's just a matter of timing.

AFTERWORD

As I mentioned, I wrote several articles about my experiences as a carer. Here are three which were published in the *Alzheimer's Disease Society Newsletter* between 1994 and 1996.

Washing-up – Then and Now

It was simple and effective, the ideal arrangement. I did the cooking. We both enjoyed the eating. My husband did the washing-up. He was useless at making meals and I was pretty awful at washing-up (although I must confess I didn't try very hard). At washing-up times I was banned from the kitchen and sat with my feet up – reading, listening to music, watching TV or just relaxing – and it was great!

The kitchen became his kingdom and he was never happier than when he was clearing, stacking, sorting, washing, rinsing, drying and putting away. And I was happy to see the results: sparkling glasses, gleaming china and cutlery, not a stain or a smear anywhere. Oh yes, it was the ideal arrangement – *then*.

But what is it like *now*? After almost 11 years of Alzheimer's Disease, what of the washing-up today? Slowly, relentlessly, the standard has deteriorated beyond recognition. Only one thing remains the same – my husband's determination to 'help'. It is the only thing he still tries to do – the only activity that makes him feel useful and helps him keep his self-esteem.

At the first rattle or clink he is there. I never cease to be amazed at this reaction, as he seems oblivious to anything else.

For me, relaxing is no longer possible as I hover in the background, pretending not to do anything but desperately trying to

136

prevent any major disasters. I must let him do it. I must help him keep his self-esteem.

At first things were not too bad. It was simply the length of time it took. Washing-up took forever and it was not unusual for him to spend most of the evening in the kitchen. But gradually the variations on a theme began. I marvel at how many permutations there are in the simple art of washing up. Simple? Never in a million years! I reckon a win on the pools is more likely than a correct prediction of my husband's washing-up methods.

Paradoxically, the worse he gets, the easier it gets for me. He is no longer shooing me out of the kitchen and I now find it possible to do most of the work myself, while letting him think he is in charge. He collects the dirty dishes. I quietly bring into the kitchen all the ones he has missed.

Sorting is a thing of the past for him. Fine china and heavy pans have a 50/50 chance of sharing the sink unless I get there first – and I make sure of that! He likes to run the water (if he can find the taps) with the result that it is sometimes hot, more often cold, sometimes with no washing-up liquid, sometimes with soapsuds up to his elbows. I make some excuse like needing to rinse something and add water to a more acceptable standard. Even better, he sometimes accepts my offer to wash while he dries. By the time I have finished he will only have dried two or three things. They will be 'stacked' – upside-down, on their sides, big dishes balanced on small ones...

I have to be particularly vigilant at this time, ready to rescue things, to make sure he doesn't pick up an unwashed item to dry and most importantly to check the cloth! He will pick up the first thing to hand – a dirty cloth, a hand towel – even on one occasion, a duster that shouldn't have been there (no comment). Thank goodness I manage to sort him out.

By this time, I am usually a bundle of nerves and he is losing interest. I take over, finish off and put everything away. He doesn't notice but when I give him a big hug and thank him for doing *all* the work, he usually smiles and walks away well pleased with himself.

I don't suppose even this stage will last for much longer. But whilst it does, and whilst he still feels important, *three cheers for washing up* say I.

Media Madness

It was all my fault! I was irritated by the BBC's 'Age Watch' questionnaire. How could I give simple answers to questions which warranted a full essay of explanation? Nevertheless, I decided to complete it, adding full explanations where necessary, sent it off and forgot it.

Months later I was approached by a BBC producer about appearing in an Esther Rantzen documentary 'Never too Late'. 'You're too late already' I thought! But gradually I was won over. I even began to think that our contribution might help to spread the word about Alzheimer's Disease and its devastating effect on sufferers and carers.

The filming would take place in October. I spent sleepless nights anticipating the questions and rehearsing my replies and got myself tied in knots, worrying. How would my husband react? What would they do to the house? How long would it take? How would I find free time to go and have a hair-do? Just what had I let myself in for?

It took two days of filming to produce an edited version of about eight minutes. But what interesting days they were! The film crew were great; it was organised chaos with cameras, lights and sound equipment everywhere. The producer's personal assistant became my PA too – I only had to say the words 'tea or coffee' and she shot off to the kitchen to make drinks for everyone. And I was immediately at ease with Esther – she was really caring and the interview went without a hitch.

I began to panic again as the date of the broadcast drew nearer. What if the whole thing was a farce and we hadn't helped the cause of people with Alzheimer's at all? After the broadcast I relaxed – perhaps it wasn't too bad after all. But then the phone calls started, and the letters, the cards, the personal callers at the house ... on and on it went! So this is what being in the limelight is all about!

One very important call came from the Alzheimer's Disease Society – would I possibly consider helping with a video? I heard myself saying 'Yes'. Well, what the heck, having done it once, there's nothing to it, is there?!

Michael Barratt was the producer this time, and there was an instant rapport between us. He showed great consideration, with more than a little understanding of what we were going through.

It was the now familiar routine. My nerves disappeared and I was completely at ease. The whole thing took just over two hours, and that included a relief break when Stan became very fidgety and had to be taken to the toilet. I am very proud of our contribution to the completed video.

Our lives have now moved onto a new stage. Stan was taken ill and admitted to hospital soon after the filming. He is now in a nursing home and I am once more trying to come to terms with this latest upheaval and all its conflicting emotions.

Now one of my most precious possessions is a copy of the whole recording we made complete with mistakes and retakes, and especially the parts where Stan tried so valiantly to find the right words. Polite as always he expressed his hopes that 'his staff' had shown them the 'whole system'. He thanked them for their visit, describing it as 'immaculate'. And, most poignant of all, he described our wonderful marriage as 'fruitful'.

I do know exactly what he means. We have had the most wonderful life together and if the making of this video provides more understanding of Alzheimer's Disease and ways of finding help, then perhaps fruitful is the right word after all.

On a Journey to Nowhere

It was 1983 when our journey began. Just my husband and I and a long, lonely journey through Alzheimer's Disease. A journey that still continues. But today the tunnels are getting much darker and the stations are greyer. There are still the two of us, but for many years I have been the only one aware of getting closer and closer to the journey's end.

It began with our early retirement when my husband was just 57. The retirement had been forced on us because of the onset of Alzheimer's Disease. 'Early retirement – you are lucky!' was the remark heard over and over again. I bit my lip and said nothing.

The journey was pleasant enough at first – days out, meals out, time to visit family and friends, time for extra holidays. We enjoyed pottering in the garden, walking, exploring and we even ventured abroad.

But gradually, imperceptibly, came the inevitable difficulties and hazards along the way. The tunnels became areas of anxiety, despair, tiredness and frustration as I watched my wonderful husband change completely. He could no longer read, write or talk coherently. He began to hallucinate and have bouts of aggression. He could do nothing for himself. Worst of all, he had occasional flashes of insight into what was happening and I felt powerless to console him.

He also began to wander. I have lost him all over the place, which must appear extremely careless of me! My worst nightmare was in London. Imagine the scene: Liverpool Street Station in the rush hour. Me, juggling with the luggage and scanning the indicator board to find the platform we needed. Stan stood by my side. Then suddenly he wasn't there, he had been swept along with the crowd and just vanished into thin air. It was the worst moment in my life. What if he got on a train, any train, going who knows where? How I spotted him I'll never know but in those few moments I died a thousand deaths. Ironically, the platform we needed was number 13 – I shan't forget that.

And all the other times he wandered off – Barafundle beach in South Wales, close to the M4 in Berkshire and on the A38 near home – thank goodness I always got him back unharmed and quite oblivious of the anxiety he had caused.

Our journey continued to be fraught with difficulties; the biggest of all for me was learning how to 'let go'. We had always done everything together and now, after 46 years of marriage, I had to learn to accept that separation was on the horizon in the form of day care, respite care and finally nursing home care. Each one took me through another tunnel, longer, darker and more difficult to negotiate than anything that had happened before.

He is now in a nursing home, well cared for by a devoted and caring staff. Somewhere along our journey, probably many years ago, I lost him. Lost to Alzheimer's Disease. He doesn't need me now. He only needs to be comfortable, warm, clean and well-fed. Other people have taken over. He registers no recognition when I visit him. There are no remaining memories.

The most quoted remark to me about him going into a home is, 'It must be like a bereavement.' I really have no way of knowing. All I know is that ever since 1983 there has been grief. It is grief without the mourning, and that is all it can be.

So where are we now? Still journeying on, still negotiating the tunnels on the bad days. Still caring. Still loving. One day, I know, the journey will end. Only then will I be able to grieve openly.

The following articles were written for the newsletter distributed from the clinical psychologist at Newtown Hospital, Worcester:

Living with Grief

We had everything anyone could wish for. A wonderful marriage, a lovely home, fulfilling jobs, gorgeous children and grand-children, mutual interests and hobbies and many happy thoughts for our future retirement.

It was too good to last! Fate, in the guise of Alzheimer's Disease, intervened – and slowly, almost imperceptibly, every-thing has changed. So many changes, so many losses along the way – and some of them so very hard to bear!

The material changes hit us first. Loss of employment for us both, then the caravan, the car, expensive holidays and outings. They affect us – of course they do – but we can get by without them, they are no longer important to us and we have adapted to life without them. Social changes too. We suffered the isolation and loneliness that inevitably happens as 'friends' drift away and forget to keep in touch. It hurts and humiliates – but new 'real' friends have taken their place and once again we have survived.

There are other losses that are so much harder to bear. How hard it is to see the one you love slowly losing all ability to do the things we take for granted. Things like washing, shaving, dressing, eat-ing. We have devised ways of coping – even laughed and joked about it all. But deep down the hurt remains and I grieve to see my dear husband reduced to such an existence. He was the practical one, but now cannot even work out how to turn on the light. He

141

had a gift for figures but is now unable to add together two plus two. He is unable to write, make sense verbally or comprehend what is said. These are the losses that really hurt.

Then there are all the downward steps he has had to take – the first time at day care, the first respite care, the registration as partially sighted. He cannot convey to me his thoughts and feelings, except by showing aggression as a way of expressing his frustration. All I know is that for me each step is another agonising loss as I feel him slipping away from me.

I feel so sad when I think of our retirement plans. He doesn't even know he *is* retired – he never has and never will fulfil any of his dreams. It's the loss of my dreams, too. I've lost my companion and my helpmate – and there is no one to turn to for comfort, no shoulder to cry on.

I look at him – so lost, so withdrawn, so vulnerable – and all I want to do is hug him and reassure him. Sometimes there is no response. Sometimes he doesn't even know me. That is the biggest loss of all.

I see what he has become. I think of what he used to be like. The sense of loss is overwhelming. A line of my poem goes round and round in my brain. 'Heartache for the man he is. Grief for what he was before'. For me, that seems to say it all.

What is a Carer?

Some time ago, I looked up the word 'carer' in my dictionary and was shocked to discover that it wasn't even listed. My edition was published in 1988 – five years *after* I became a carer. I sincerely hope that later editions are now acknowledging that carers do exist and are playing vital rôles in today's society. The word 'care' was there, of course. And 'caretakers' and 'careworkers' got a mention, as did expressions such as 'Who cares?', 'couldn't care less' and 'for all I care'. People could be 'carefree' or 'careworn', but *not* 'carers'.

I delved deeper. The old English word was 'caru' – a noun meaning 'trouble or sorrow', or a verb meaning 'to grieve'. Today, however, care implies some degree of control. We have 'care and 'protection' of juveniles which may lead to a 'care order' or being 'placed in care'. In 1990 we had the 'Community Care Act' with rules for long-term provision for the elderly. I wonder if those rules still apply? Today, all the talk is of 'Care in the Community', which sounds fine, but in reality it means the closure of psychiatric hospitals, the disappearance of long-stay beds and the closing down of many state-maintained nursing homes. For whatever reason 'Care in the Community' is simply not working.

The adjective 'caring' is much used. We now have a whole army of caring professionals – health workers, social workers, doctors, nurses, teachers, therapists etc. – all part of our 'caring society'. They are, for the most part, dedicated and very hard-working. But at the end of their working day they can go home and at the end of the month they can collect their pay cheque.

Not so the 'carers' with their own very personal problems and responsibilities. For many, their caring goes on unrecognised all day, every day and seemingly forever.

So back to the question, 'What is a carer?' I can only give you my own personal answer, not a dictionary definition. When people ask me what it is like, my answers are many and varied – perhaps because the questioners are also many and varied. Often, all I need to say is that being a carer is a difficult and tiring job. No more explanation is necessary and the questioner is satisfied. But not always. Sometimes I have to dig deep and search for the reality. I have to tell them of my mental and physical tiredness, of the emotional upheavals and the demands on all my reserves. I have to admit to the stress and consequent health problems, to the social deprivation and the feeling of isolation. And I have to tell them of the anguish I feel as I watch the person I love go through the ever downward mental, physical, behavioural and personality changes which will ultimately be fatal.

I try to tell them all these things. They may nod sympatheti-cally. They may be genuine in their offers of help. But always, I am left with the same feeling and the same thought – that they can-not possibly comprehend what it is really like.

In March 1995, after 12 years of caring, my husband reached the stage when it became impossible for me to look after him on my own, and with much heart-searching, I reluctantly arranged nursing home care for him. My physical tiredness has disappeared and I now have some free time, but in all respects I am still the same. I am still very much a carer. Only other carers will understand and will be truly sympathetic. To them I say, 'God bless and take care.'